MW00876292

Epigraph

Acquired immunity is a system that learns to recognize a pathogen. When a foreign substance enters the body, these cells and organs create antibodies and lead to multiplication of immune cells that are specific to that harmful substance and attack and destroy it. Our immune system then adapts by remembering the foreign substance so that if it enters again, these antibodies and cells are even more efficient and quick to destroy it.

— Harvard T.H. Chan Medical School of
Public Health

[Harvard T.H. Chan Medical School of Public Health. (2022). *Nutrition and Immunity*. Harvard T.H. Chan Medical School of Public Health: Boston, Massachusetts. Retrieved 3 July 2022 https://www.hsph.harvard.edu/nutritionsource/nutrition-and-immunity/]

Contents

Part III: Transmission and Prevalence of HPV

Part IV: Treatment of Cervical Dysplasia

Part V: Diagnosis and Treatment of Warts

Part VI: Men and HPV

Part VII: HPV-associated Conditions

Prologue

o you need information about HPV, Pap smears, cervical dysplasia, and warts?

This book will provide the essential facts about them. You will learn critical information about HPV diagnosis and treatment.

We will evaluate various treatments of HPV, determine how to treat it effectively, and how best to develop immunity to it.

This book will provide facts about these topics.

- HPV diagnosis, transmission, treatments, and immunity.
- Cervical dysplasia diagnosis and treatments.
- Warts diagnosis and treatments.

- HPV risks for infertility, miscarriages, pregnancy, and cervical cancer.
- Oral HPV, anal HPV, urethritis, and vaginosis.
- HPV risks for penile cancer and prostate disease.

We will cover these seven Parts and topics.

Part I: Fundamentals of HPV and Cervical Dysplasia. The natural history of HPV, immunology of HPV, HPV types, HPV reinfection, and cervical cancer.

Part II: Diagnosis of HPV and Cervical Dysplasia. Pap smear screening, limitations of ASCUS Pap smears, self-sampling for HPV, degrees of cervical dysplasia, colposcopy and biopsy, and HPV false-negative results.

Part III: Transmission and Prevalence of HPV. HPV transmission in general, HPV transmission during childbirth, cervical dysplasia during pregnancy, and prevalence and public awareness of HPV.

Part IV: Treatment of Cervical Dysplasia. Medical treatments of trichloroacetic acid and 5-fluorouracil; surgical treatments of LEEP, cone biopsy, and cryotherapy; alternative treatments of beta-carotene, folic acid, vitamin C, indole-3-carbinol, AHCC, and Beta-mannan™; the value of *Aloe vera* and iodine as critical supports for the immune system to prevent and treat infections.

Part V: Diagnosis and Treatment of Warts. Genital, plantar, palmar, flat, and common warts; medical, surgical, and alternative treatments; conditions that may be confused with warts such as pearly penile papules and molluscum contagiosum.

Part VI: Men and HPV. HPV-related diseases in men such as penile cancer, prostate disease, and prostate cancer.

Part VII: HPV-associated Conditions. Infertility, miscarriages, oral lesions, anal cancer, urethritis, vaginosis, vulvar vestibulitis syndrome, lichen sclerosus, and skin tags.

Part I: Fundamentals of HPV and Cervical Dysplasia

Chapter 1
Natural History of Human Papillomavirus Infection

H PV is an acronym for "Human PapillomaVirus."

When Pap smears detect mild abnormalities in cervical cells, the results show what the medical community calls low-grade squamous intraepithelial lesions, also called LGSIL, LSIL, CIN-1, or mild dysplasia.

LGSIL (and LSIL) are acronyms for "Low-Grade Squamous Intraepithelial Lesion." The low-grade lesions may also be described as caused by LR, or "Low-Risk," HPV types.

CIN is an acronym for "Cervical Intraepithelial Neoplasia."

When Pap smears detect moderate or severe abnormalities in cervical cells, they are called high-grade squamous intraepithelial lesions, also called HGSIL, HSIL, CIN-2, CIN-3, or moderate to severe dysplasia.

HGSIL (and HSIL) are acronyms for "**High-G**rade **S**quamous **I**ntraepithelial **L**esion." The high-grade lesions may also be described as caused by HR, or "**High-Risk**," HPV types.

It will be helpful to know these classifications when you read about various HPV studies.

These classifications are usually determined initially by a Pap smear. This is an examination of cervical cells and also referred to as cervical cytology.

We will present medical evidence that you can develop immunity to HPV and eliminate it.

Not everyone is convinced that HPV can be eliminated. But before evaluating treatments, let's first look at the normal progression of HPV without treatment.

The normal progression of any untreated disease is described as its "natural history." Any treatment must be compared to this to determine its value.

Any worthwhile disease remedy should have a higher cure rate than what would naturally happen without treatment.

The natural history of HPV shows clearance in 51.9% of women within one year.

Dr. John Sellors and eight medical colleagues at the Department of Family Medicine at McMaster University in Hamilton Ontario Canada published an article in the February 2003 issue of the *Canadian Medical Association Journal.* It has been cited as authoritative in over 60 medical articles. Dr. Sellors stated: "Of the previously HPV-positive women, 51.9% had cleared the infection. A large proportion of the women who were HPV-positive appeared to have cleared the infection after one year."

[Sellors, J.W., et al. (2003). Incidence, clearance, and predictors of human papillomavirus infection in women. *CMAJ. 2003 Feb 18; 168 (4): 421-5.* https:// pubmed.ncbi.nlm.nih.gov/12591782/]

The natural history of HPV shows clearance in 70% of young women within two years.

Studies of the natural history of HPV show that *even when untreated,* 70% of young women with HPV develop immunity and a negative HPV test within 24 months. This landmark study by Dr. Anna-Barbara Moscicki has been cited in over 100 medical articles. This is a strong testimony to the value of the study.

Dr. Moscicki and twelve medical colleagues at the Department of Pediatrics of the University of California Medical School in San Francisco California published this article in the February 1998 issue of the *Journal of Pediatrics.* Dr. Moscicki said:

The objectives of this study were to describe the early natural history of human papillomavirus infection by examining a cohort of young women positive for an HPV test. 618 women positive for HPV participated. HPV testing, cytologic evaluation, and colposcopic evaluation were performed at 4-month intervals. Approximately 70% of women were found to have HPV regression by 24 months. Women with low-risk HPV type infections were more likely to show HPV regression than were women with high-risk HPV type infections.

Dr. Moscicki summarized:

Most young women with a positive HPV test will become negative within a 24-month period. However, we found that most young women with persistent positive HPV tests did not have cytologically perceptible HSIL over a 2-year period.

[Moscicki, A.B., et al. (1998). The natural history of human papillomavirus infection as measured by repeated DNA testing in adolescents and young women. *J Pediatr. 1998 Feb; 132 (2): 277-84.* https:// pubmed.ncbi.nlm.nih.gov/9506641/]

The natural history of HPV shows clearance in

61% of young women within one year and clearance in 91% within three years.

Dr. Moscicki and ten medical colleagues at the Department of Pediatrics of the University of California Medical School in San Francisco California published an article in the November 2004 issue of the *Lancet* journal. It focused on the regression of low-grade squamous intraepithelial lesions. The study included 187 female adolescents with LSIL, aged 13-22 years, who were examined every four months by cytology, colposcopy, and HPV test. Regression was defined as at least three consecutive normal Pap smears. The regression probability was 61% at 12 months and 91% at 36 months of follow-up. Dr. Moscicki concluded:

> The high rate of regression recorded in this study lends support to observation by cytology in the management of LSIL in female adolescents. Negative HPV status was associated with regression, suggesting that HPV testing could be helpful in monitoring LSIL.

[Moscicki, A.B., et al. (2004). Regression of low-grade squamous intra-epithelial lesions in young women. *Lancet. 2004 Nov 6-12; 364 (9446): 1678-83.* https://pubmed.ncbi.nlm.nih.gov/15530628/]

The fact that HPV can be eliminated should

encourage those who have this infection. HPV does not always disappear within two years *when left untreated*, but in most cases, HPV immunity is acquired within two years.

The natural history of cutaneous HPV warts shows clearance in 50% of children within one year.

Dr. Sjoerd Bruggink and five medical colleagues at the Leiden University Medical Center in Leiden Netherlands published an article in the September 2013 issue of the *Annals of Family Medicine* journal. It concerned the natural history of cutaneous HPV warts in over 1,000 primary school children. Dr. Bruggink reported that one-half of primary school children were free of warts within one year without any treatment and concluded:

> Patients and Family Physicians should weigh the benign natural course, the adverse effects of treatments, and the costs on the one hand, and the effectiveness of treatments and the risk of spreading untreated warts on the other.

[Bruggink, S.C., et al. (2013). Natural course of cutaneous warts among primary school children: a prospective cohort study. *Ann Fam Med. 2013 Sep; 11 (5): 437–441.* https://pubmed.ncbi.nlm.nih.gov/24019275/]

The natural history for clearance of HPV is 50-61% within one year, 70% within two years, and 91% within three years. The effectiveness of any treatment should be compared to these natural history results.

It is essential for optimal health to understand what treatments can accelerate the development of immunity. We will cover these in detail.

Various non-surgical and herbal treatments can accelerate the clearance of HPV and help develop immunity to it. Even some types of surgery can have a secondary effect of doing this as well.

Immunity to HPV is acquired frequently.

Immunity to HPV must specify a particular HPV type - one of the 228 currently identified genotypes. If a person tests positive for a particular type or types, but later tests negative for them, then that person has achieved immunity for those particular types, assuming the test result is not a false-negative result.

HPV-negative tests do not rule out an HPV infection because (1) less than 10% of the known 228 HPV types are usually tested, and (2) the tests can yield false-negative results even for the few types tested. Therefore, treatment may be considered if HPV is suspected in the presence of HPV symptoms in the patient or the patient's partner.

Chapter 2
Immunology of HPV

There are many viruses to which we readily develop immunity. These include the over 300 cold viruses, as well as measles, mumps, chickenpox, and even HPV.

However, HPV and several other viruses manage to avoid the immune system in some people. They avoid the humoral and cellular immune responses, the B-cells and the T-cells, respectively. But when immunity to an HPV type does occur, the body is no longer infected or contagious for that type. As a result of immunity, the signs and symptoms clear, and the same HPV type can no longer infect the individual.

HPV may evade detection by the immune system.

Dr. Margaret Stanley at the University of Cambridge

in Cambridge England published an article in the October 1998 issue of the *European Journal of Dermatology*. She reviewed the evidence of immune evasion by HPV in genital warts. Dr. Stanley said:

> Such findings suggest that the immune system is ignorant or indifferent to the infection. Evidence from regressing genital warts in humans and animal models suggests that HPV is a cell-mediated immune response.

[Stanley, M. (1998). The immunology of genital human papillomavirus infection. *Eur J Dermatol. Oct-Nov 1998; 8 (7 Suppl): 8-12; discussion 20-2.* https://pubmed.ncbi.nlm.nih.gov/10387957/]

Naturally-acquired HPV antibodies offer protection against subsequent infection from the same HPV type.

Dr. Xingmei Yao at the National Institute of Diagnostics of Xiamen University in Fujian China, and thirty medical colleagues, published an article in the July 2021 issue of the *Lancet Regional Health West Pacific* journal. It concerned naturally-acquired immunity for HPV and included 3,634 women aged 18-45 years. These doctors found that naturally-acquired antibodies for HPV reduced the risk of reinfection for the same HPV type.

Dr. Yao said: "Naturally-acquired antibodies are associated with a substantially reduced risk of subsequent homotypic infection."

[Yao, X., et al. (2021). Naturally acquired HPV antibodies against subsequent homotypic infection: A large-scale prospective cohort study. *Lancet Reg Health West Pac. 2021 Aug; 13: 100196.* https://pubmed.ncbi.nlm.nih.gov/34527987/]

Immunity to HPV is acquired frequently.

Immunity to HPV must specify a particular HPV type - one of the 228 currently identified. If a person tests positive for a particular type or types, but later tests negative for them, then that person has achieved immunity for those particular types, assuming the test result is not a false-negative result.

HPV-negative tests do not rule out an HPV infection because (1) less than 10% of the known 228 HPV types are usually tested, and (2) the tests can yield false-negative results even for the few types tested. Therefore, treatment may be considered if HPV is suspected in the presence of HPV symptoms in the patient or the patient's partner.

Chapter 3
HPV Type Associations

When the medical community speaks of the HPV virus, it is essential to know that HPV refers to a group of 228 related viruses. This means they have a very similar but not identical genetic code. Also, not all have the same risks or effects. These 228 variants of HPV are numbered as *types* such as type 1, 2, etc. Various studies will often refer to the particular HPV types relevant to the disease discussed.

HPV was detected in 21.8% of asymptomatic female college students, of which 11.8% had high-risk HPV types such as types 16, 18, 31, and 45.

Dr. H. Richardson and five medical colleagues at the Department of Oncology of McGill University in Montreal Canada published an article in the February 2000 issue of the journal of *Sexually Transmitted Diseases*. Dr.

Richardson studied the prevalence of HPV infection in asymptomatic women and reported:

> The overall HPV prevalence was 21.8%. A low-risk HPV infection was found in 6.2% of the women; 11.8% had a high-risk HPV infection with types 16, 18, 31, 33, 35, 39, 45, 51, 52, 56, and 58; 7.1% had an unknown HPV type; and 2.7% had a multiple type infection.

[Richardson, H., et al. (2000). Determinants of low-risk and high-risk cervical human papillomavirus infections in Montreal University students. *Sex Transm Dis. 2000 Feb; 27 (2): 79-86.* https://pubmed.ncbi.nlm.nih.gov/10676974/]

Some HPV types have a significant association with cervical dysplasia and cervical cancer.

The HPV types most commonly associated with CIN 2-3 and cervical cancer are types 16, 18, 31, and 45.

Dr. Efraim Siegler at the Department of Obstetrics and Gynecology of Carmel Medical Center in Haifa Israel, and six medical colleagues, published an article in the June 2017 issue of the *Minerva Ginecologica* journal. They identified the HPV types most often associated with CIN-2, CIN-3, and cervical cancer. Dr. Siegler said:

In the CIN 2-3 group, the most common HPV types were 16, 31, and 18, and in the cancer group HPV 16, 45, and 18. Multiple HPV types were seen in 12.8% of the CIN 2-3 group but only in 0.9% of the cancer group.

[Siegler, E., et al. (2017). The prevalence of HPV types in women with CIN 2-3 or cervical cancer in Haifa District, Israel. *Minerva Ginecol. 2017 Jun; 69 (3): 211-217.* https://pubmed.ncbi.nlm.nih.gov/27636902/]

Dr. P.L. Cheah and Dr. L.M. Looi at the Department of Pathology of the Faculty of Medicine of the University of Malaya in Kuala Lumpur Malaysia published an article in the June 1998 issue of the *Malaysia Journal of Pathology*. Dr. Cheah noted that HPV types described in cervical lesions are categorized into high-risk types and low-risk types.

Skin warts are usually associated with HPV types 1, 2, 3, 7, and 10. Genital warts are usually associated with HPV types 6 and 11.

Genital warts are also called anogenital warts, condyloma acuminata, vaginal warts, penile warts, verruca acuminata, or venereal warts.

HPV types 6 and 11 are the same HPV types seen in recurrent juvenile laryngeal papillomas and are probably transmitted by passage through the birth canal.

Nasal cavity lesions generally have HPV types of 6,

11, and 57. Oral cavity HPV lesions generally have types 6, 11, 13, and 32. Warty lip lesions are generally HPV type 2. Conjunctival papillomas of the eye are usually HPV types 6 and 11.

[Cheah, P.L., et al. (1998). Biology and pathological associations of the human papillomaviruses: a review. *Malays J Pathol. 1998 Jun; 20 (1): 1-10.* https://pubmed. ncbi.nlm.nih.gov/10879257/]

HPV-negative tests do not rule out an HPV infection because (1) less than 10% of the known 228 HPV types are usually tested, and (2) the tests can yield false-negative results even for the few types tested. Therefore, treatment may be considered if HPV is suspected in the presence of HPV symptoms in the patient or the patient's partner.

Chapter 4
HPV Reinfection and Carrier States

S ome believe that HPV remains in a carrier state for years, but this is probably uncommon.

As I've mentioned, there are 228 HPV types. This may be the reason some believe that long carrier states are standard. What may be viewed as an HPV carrier state may simply be subsequent infections by different HPV types over the years.

The number of identified HPV types is 228 and increasing.

Dr. Babban Jee at the Department of Health Research of the Ministry of Health and Family Welfare in New Delhi India, and three medical colleagues, published an article in the August 2021 issue of the *International Reviews of Immunology* journal. Dr. Jee said: "To date, 228 genotypes of HPV have been identified."

[Jee, B., et al. (2021). Immunology of HPV-mediated cervical cancer: current understanding. *Int Rev Immunol. 2021; 40 (5): 359-378.* https://pubmed.ncbi. nlm.nih.gov/32853049/]

There are over 300 common cold viruses, yet no one considers the common cold virus to be in a perpetual carrier state that flares up periodically. The same situation applies to HPV.

There is very little cross-immunity among the different HPV types. This means that if someone has immunity to one HPV type, that specific immunity is usually not effective against another HPV type.

A different HPV type can likely infect a person immune to some other HPV types. This is not reinfection since the new HPV infection is a different HPV type.

HPV can be compared to the common cold because immunity to one cold virus does not protect a person against all the other cold viruses. But as a person has more colds, there are fewer colds for that person to catch. Young children average ten colds yearly, whereas adults average only three colds yearly because adults have developed immunity for many cold viruses.

Immunity to HPV is acquired frequently.

Immunity to HPV must specify a particular HPV type - one of the 228 currently identified. If a person tests positive for a particular type or types, but later tests negative for them, then that person has achieved immunity for those particular types, assuming the test result is not a false-negative result.

Again, HPV-negative tests do not rule out an HPV infection because (1) less than 10% of the known 228 HPV types are usually tested, and (2) the tests can yield false-negative results even for the few types tested. Therefore, treatment may be considered if HPV is suspected in the presence of HPV symptoms in the patient or the patient's partner.

Chapter 5
Cervical Cancer

Cervical dysplasia and cervical cancer are believed to be caused by HPV in over 99% of the cases. Moreover, HPV is the only proven cause of cervical dysplasia, cervical cancer, and warts. But HPV may not always be detected, even when present, due to false-negative test results.

HPV is the accepted primary cause of cervical cancer.

Dr. C. Meg McLachlin at the London Health Sciences Center of the University of Western Ontario in Ontario Canada published an article in the June 2000 issue of the *Clinics of Laboratory Medicine* journal. The report made it clear that there is significant evidence linking HPV to cervical cancer. Dr. McLachlin states: "HPV is now accepted as the primary cause of cervical neoplasia and accounts for most of the risk factors traditionally associated with this disease."

[McLachlin, C.M. (2000). Human papillomavirus in cervical neoplasia: role, risk factors, and implications. *Clin Lab Med 2000 Jun; 20 (2): 257-70.* https://pubmed. ncbi.nlm.nih.gov/10863640/]

Even as early as 1993, it was established that HPV caused most cervical dysplasia.

Cervical cancer is linked mainly to the high-risk HPV types.

Dr. Mark H. Schiffman at the Epidemiology and Biostatistics Program of the National Cancer Institute in Bethesda Maryland, and eleven medical colleagues, published an article in the June 1993 issue of the *Journal of the National Cancer Institute*. Over 200 medical articles cited it. Dr. Schiffman noted: "The data show that the great majority of all grades of cervical dysplasia can be attributed to HPV infection, particularly with the cancer-associated types of HPV."

[Schiffman, M.H., et al. (1993). Epidemiologic evidence showing that human papillomavirus infection causes most cervical intraepithelial neoplasia. *J Natl Cancer Inst. 1993 Jun 16; 85 (12): 958-64.* https:// pubmed.ncbi.nlm.nih.gov/8388478/]

HPV was found in 99.7% of cervical cancers.

Dr. Nubia Munoz at the International Agency for

Research on Cancer in Lyon France published an article in the October 2000 issue of the *Journal of Clinical Virology*. It has been cited in over 100 medical publications. It stated that 99.7% of 1,000 cases of cervical cancer in 22 countries were shown to be HPV-positive. HPV types 16 and 18 were most commonly found, followed by types 31, 33, and 45. The second set of studies discussed by Dr. Munoz was conducted in 13 countries that included 2,000 cases. The following types can also be carcinogenic: HPV 35, 51, 52, 58, and 59. As Dr. Munoz summarizes: "Our studies provide the most solid epidemiological evidence to conclude that HPV is not only the central cause of cervical cancer worldwide but also a necessary cause."

[Munoz, N. (2000). Human papillomavirus and cancer: the epidemiological evidence. *J Clin Virol. 2000 Oct; 19 (1-2): 1-5.* https://pubmed.ncbi.nlm.nih.gov/11091143/]

There is compelling evidence that HPV is the cause of cervical cancer; this belief is now widely accepted.

Chapter 6
Rarity of CIN-1 Progression to CIN-3

C ervical dysplasia progression to cervical cancer usually takes several years, if it occurs at all. Progression normally does not happen. However, the likelihood of progression is determined by many factors, including, most importantly, HPV type and the status of the immune system of the individual.

Low-grade dysplasia (CIN-1) rarely progresses to high-grade dysplasia (CIN-3).

Dr. Clare Gilham at the London School of Hygiene and Tropical Medicine in London England, and three medical colleagues, published an article in the June 2019 issue of the *Health Technology Assessment* journal. Dr. Gilham said:

About three-quarters of women with HPV infection and normal cytology clear their infections within about 3 years. Their risk of CIN-3+ within this time frame is low (1.5%), suggesting that the current policy of annual repeat testing and referral after 2 years may be unnecessarily cautious. Approximately 40% of women who remained HPV+ had cleared their initial infection and acquired a new HPV type. The cumulative CIN-3+ risks in women with type-specific persistent infections are about six times higher than in women with new infections. Triage strategies based on HPV persistence would, therefore, reduce unnecessary referral of women with new (and largely transient) infections.

[Gilham, C., et al. (2019). HPV testing compared with routine cytology in cervical screening: long-term follow-up of ARTISTIC RCT. *Health Technol Assess. 2019 Jun; 23 (28): 1-44.* https://pubmed.ncbi.nlm.nih.gov/31219027/]

CIN-1 may progress to CIN-3 in 1.5% of cases but CIN-1 shows clearance of 80% within 3-4 years.

Dr. Maria Teresa Bruno at the Department of General Surgery of the University of Catania in Catania Italy, and three medical colleagues, published an article in the March 2021 issue of the journal of *Infectious*

Diseases of Obstetrics and Gynecology. They studied the possible progression of CIN-1 to CIN-3. Dr. Bruno noted that CIN-1 would spontaneously regress in 80% of the cases. Some doctors believe that CIN-1 can progress to CIN-3 in 10% of the cases.

In this study, only 1.5% of the CIN-1 patients developed CIN-3 within four years. Dr. Bruno concluded:

> The most likely explanations for progression from LSIL to HSIL are (1) actual progression, (2) under-diagnosis of HSIL on initial biopsy, (3) over-diagnosis of HSIL on follow-up biopsy or cone, and (4) CIN-3 arose de novo. Analyzing the histological exams of the cones of the 7 cases that progressed to high-grade, we found the coexistence of CIN-1 and CIN-3 lesions in all cases. Some recent studies have shown that a viral genotype corresponds to different lesions in the same cervix; therefore, CIN-1 coexisting with CIN-3 does not always indicate the progression of CIN-1. Other authors have doubted the capacity of LSIL to progress.

[Bruno, M.T., et al. (2021). Progression of CIN-1/LSIL HPV persistent of the cervix: actual progression or CIN-3 coexistence. *Infect Dis Obstet Gynecol. 2021 Mar 9; 2021: 6627531.* https://pubmed.ncbi.nlm.nih.gov/33776406/]

Chapter 7
Abnormal Pap Smears after Hysterectomy

A bnormal Pap smears indicate that vaginal dysplasia can occur following a hysterectomy, but this is very uncommon and occurs in less than 3% of hysterectomies. In cases of hysterectomy, the Pap smear is taken from the vaginal cuff and is called a vaginal Pap smear, vaginal cuff smear, vaginal cuff cytology, vaginal smear, or vaginal cytology.

Pap smears are not recommended after hysterectomies for non-cancerous cervical conditions in HPV-negative patients.

Dr. Joanne T. Piscitelli and three medical colleagues at the Division of General Obstetrics and Gynecology of Duke University in Durham North Carolina published an article in the August 1995 issue of the *American Journal of Obstetrics and Gynecology*. These doctors completed a 10-year follow-up of 697 women who had undergone hysterectomy for non-cancerous reasons. Dr. Piscitelli said:

> We needed 633 tests to detect one true positive case of vaginal dysplasia. The low incidence of vaginal dysplasia and carcinoma, combined with the high false-positive rate, supports decreasing the number of screening tests performed for these low-risk patients.

[Piscitelli, J.T., et al. (1995). Cytologic screening after hysterectomy for benign disease. *Am J Obstet Gynecol.* 1995 Aug; 173 (2): 424-30; discussion 430-2. https://pubmed.ncbi.nlm.nih.gov/7645617/]

Dr. M.D. Fetters and two medical colleagues at the Department of Family Practice of the University of Michigan in Ann Arbor Michigan published an article in the March 1996 issue of the *Journal of the American Medical Association*. They studied the Pap smear results following total hysterectomy for non-cancerous disease. Dr. Fetters concluded: "There is insufficient evidence to recommend routine vaginal smear screening in women after total hysterectomy for benign disease."

[Fetters, M.D., et al. (1996). Effectiveness of vaginal Papanicolaou smear screening after total hysterectomy for benign disease. *JAMA. 1996 Mar 27; 275 (12): 940-7.* https://pubmed.ncbi.nlm.nih.gov/8598623/]

Dr. Andrea Videlefsky and five medical colleagues at the Department of Family Medicine of Emory University School of Medicine in Atlanta Georgia published an article in the July 2000 issue of the *Journal of the American Board of Family Practice.* The article studied the need for routine Pap smears following a hysterectomy performed for benign conditions, not performed for cervical cancer. In this study, 220 women were randomly selected for the study. 97% of 220 women observed for an average of 89 months had no HPV on vaginal cuff smears. No invasive carcinomas were found. Dysplastic lesions were detected in 3%. However, 70% had one or more infections. These infections included bacterial vaginosis, trichomoniasis, candidiasis, HPV, and herpes. Dr. Videlefsky said: "Most routine vaginal cuff cytology screening tests need not be performed in women who have had a hysterectomy for benign uterine conditions."

[Videlefsky, A., et al. (2000). Routine vaginal cuff smear testing in post-hysterectomy patients with benign uterine conditions: when is it indicated? *J Am Board Fam Pract. Jul-Aug 2000; 13 (4): 233-8.* https://pubmed.ncbi.nlm.nih.gov/10933286/]

Dr. F. Nicolas and five medical colleagues at Service

de Gynécologie in Anne-de-Bretagne France published an article in the March 2013 issue of the journal of *Gynécologie Obstétrique Fertilité & Sénologie*. They studied the need for vaginal Pap smears following total hysterectomy and found that vaginal Pap smears after endometrial cancer can be eliminated. However, Dr. Nicolas said:

> When hysterectomy is proposed as part of cervical intraepithelial neoplasia, the risk of vaginal recurrence of HPV-induced pathology fully justifies annual monitoring since recurrences or virus-induced lesions are seen up to 25 years after surgery. Finally, after hysterectomy for benign uterine non-HPV-induced, there is no need to propose a systematic follow-up cytology.

[Nicolas, F., et al. (2013). Are vaginal Pap smears necessary after total hysterectomy for CIN-3? *Gynecol Obstet Fertil. 2013 Mar; 41 (3): 196-200.* https://pubmed. ncbi.nlm.nih.gov/23499311/]

These so-called recurrences of cervical dysplasia seen for up to 25 years after hysterectomy are likely new HPV infections from a different genotype, not the original genotype.

Part II: Diagnosis of HPV and Cervical Dysplasia

Chapter 8
Pap Smear Screening

A Pap smear is a screening tool that examines cervical cells. It is also called cervical cytology. A swab is scraped across the cervix during a Pap exam to collect loose cervical cells as specimens. Some cells may appear to have an HPV infection under the microscope because HPV-infected cells have a characteristic appearance.

About 3.8% of the annual 50 million Pap smears in the USA are abnormal.

Dr. Christopher Mayer and a medical colleague at the Albany Medical College in Albany New York published an article in the January 2022 issue of the *StatPearls* journal. Dr. Mayer said:

Guidelines for Pap smear testing frequency vary between the United States Preventative Service Task Force and the American College of Obstetricians and Gynecologists but is recommended for women between the ages of 21 and 65. Screening is not a recommendation under the age of 21. The prevalence of abnormal Pap smears is around 3.8%. At least 50 million Pap smears are performed yearly. In 2019, there were an estimated 13,000 females diagnosed with cervical cancer and 4,000 females who died from cervical cancer.

[Mayer, C., et al. (2022). Abnormal Papanicolaou Smear. Treasure Island, Florida: *StatPearls Publishing. January 7, 2022.* https://www.ncbi.nlm.nih.gov/books/NBK560850/]

If two Paps are taken within a short time, the second Pap may appear normal because there will be fewer loose abnormal cells to scrape off for examination. For this reason, it is best to wait a couple of weeks between Paps. A colposcopy and biopsy may also appear normal if a recent Pap has scraped off all the abnormal cells, particularly if the dysplasia was mild or very localized.

Short intervals between Pap smears tended to show a milder result in the second Pap; however,

the time interval was less of a factor in determining the result of the second Pap than the specific pathologist evaluating it.

Dr. Theresa M. Kolben at the Department for Obstetrics and Gynecology of the Ludwig-Maximilians University in Munich Germany, and nine medical colleagues, published an article in the June 2017 issue of the journal of *Archives of Gynecology and Obstetrics*. They studied the effect of a short interval between Pap smears. Dr. Kolben reports:

> A repeat Pap smear is sometimes necessary after a short time interval or even immediately, when patients seek a second opinion or due to study participation. Most institutions, therefore, practice a minimum time span of 6-8 weeks before obtaining a second smear since a short interval is commonly believed to be associated with an increase of false-negative results in the second smear.

The subjectivity and complexity of reading Pap smears necessitate using HPV tests.

In Dr. Kolben's study, two Pap smears obtained during a short period were done for 81 women. Four different pathologists graded the results. It appeared that the length of time between Pap smears did tend to show a milder result in the second Pap; however, the time interval had less significance than the specific pathologist evaluating the Pap smear.

[Kolben, T.M., et al. (2017). Short interval between two Pap smears: effect on the result of the second smear? A prospective randomized trial. *Arch Gynecol Obstet. 2017 Jun; 295 (6): 1427-1433.* https://pubmed. ncbi.nlm.nih.gov/28405743/]

The average Pap smear slide contains 50,000 to 300,000 cells that must be examined - so a few abnormal cells within a crowded background of healthy cells can be missed, particularly by overworked doctors. False-negative rates of 20-30% have been reported for Pap smears.

Dr. Eileen M. Burd at the Department of Pathology of Henry Ford Hospital in Detroit Michigan published an article in the January 2003 issue of the *Clinical Microbiology Reviews* journal about HPV and cervical cancer. Dr. Burd said:

The Pap smear procedure has some limitations. Inadequate samples constitute about 8% of specimens received. False-negative rates as high as 20-30% have been reported. False-negative results can occur from the clumping of cells when the cells are not spread evenly and uniformly on the microscope slide. Some-

40

times, other contents of the cervical specimen, such as blood, bacteria, or yeast contaminate the sample and prevent the detection of abnormal cells. If exposed to air too long before being fixed on the slide, cervical cells can become distorted. Human error is probably the primary threat to accurate interpretation. The average Pap smear slide contains 50,000 to 300,000 cells that must be examined. If the sample contains only a few abnormal cells within a crowded background of healthy cells, the abnormal cells can be missed, particularly by overworked readers. In 1988, the Clinical Laboratory Improvement Act established national guidelines that restricted technicians from reading more than 100 slides per day. Some experts think that this number is still too large. Also, CLIA mandated a manual rescreening of 10% of negative satisfactory smears to reduce the number of false-negative results.

[Burd, E.M. (2003). Human papillomavirus and cervical cancer. *Clin Microbiol Rev. 2003 Jan; 16 (1): 1–17.* https://www.ncbi.nlm.nih.gov/pmc/articles/ PMC145302/]

Chapter 9
Limitations of Relying on ASCUS Pap Smears Alone

ASCUS is an acronym for Pap smears with "Atypical Squamous Cells of Undetermined Significance," which are mildly abnormal Pap smears.

There is a lack of objective results when reading ASCUS Pap smears.

One interesting study explains the problem concerning the subjectivity of reading ASCUS Paps. This further emphasizes the value of HPV testing. Notice in the following study with 200 Paps first diagnosed as ASCUS; there was very little agreement on the diagnosis when reevaluated. Five pathologists who reviewed the 200 Paps agreed on only 29%, and not a single slide was diagnosed as ASCUS by all five pathology doctors.

Dr. Mark E. Sherman and nine medical colleagues

at the Department of Pathology of Johns Hopkins Medical Center in Baltimore Maryland published an article in the August 1994 issue of the *American Journal of Clinical Pathology*. Dr. Sherman reported that five pathologists diagnosed 200 Pap smears as ASCUS, and the results were compared. Dr. Sherman said: "Exact five-way cytologic agreement was achieved in only 29% of smears, and no slide was diagnosed as atypical squamous cells of undetermined significance, or ASCUS, by all reviewers."

[Sherman, M.E., et al. (1994). Toward objective quality assurance in cervical cytopathology. Correlation of cytopathologic diagnoses with detection of high-risk human papillomavirus types. *Am J Clin Pathol. 1994 Aug; 102 (2): 182-7.* https://pubmed.ncbi.nlm.nih.gov/8042586/]

Pathologists often disagree in their evaluations of ASCUS Pap smears.

Dr. R.T. Grenko and four medical colleagues at the Department of Pathology of Penn State University College of Medicine in Hershey Pennsylvania published an article in the November 2000 issue of the *American Journal of Clinical Pathology*. The study aimed to determine whether the variability in dysplasia rates in cases of atypical squamous cells of undetermined significance also reflects variability in the interpretation of cervical biopsy specimens. Dr. Grenko said:

> 124 biopsy specimens obtained because of a cytologic diagnosis of ASCUS were reviewed independently by 5 experienced pathologists. All pathologists agreed in 28% of cases. In 52% of cases, the diagnoses ranged from benign to dysplasia. The overall interobserver agreement was poor. Agreement was better in biopsies performed for HSIL and LSIL compared to those for ASCUS. Intra-observer reproducibility in the interpretation of biopsies performed for ASCUS ranged from poor to excellent.

[Grenko, R.T., et al. (2000). Variance in the interpretation of cervical biopsy specimens obtained for atypical squamous cells of undetermined significance. *Am J Clin Pathol*. 2000 Nov; 114 (5): 735-40. https://pubmed.ncbi.nlm.nih.gov/11068547/]

The uncertain interpretations of ASCUS Pap smears or abnormal cervical biopsies suggest this. Suppose an HPV test is negative in the presence of an ASCUS Pap smear or an abnormal cervical biopsy. In that case, neither the Pap smear nor the biopsy should be relied upon to decide on treatment since the chance of having an HPV infection with a high-risk type is inconclusive.

Colposcopy and biopsy are not recommended for ASCUS Pap smears if the patient is negative for high-risk HPV types.

Dr. Eileen M. Burd at the Department of Pathology of Henry Ford Hospital in Detroit Michigan published an article in the January 2003 issue of *Clinical Microbiology Reviews* journal.

For management of ASCUS Pap smears, Dr. Burd recommended HPV testing and said:

It has been established that there is variation in interpretation of ASCUS Pap smears even among expert cytopathologists. In some women, ASCUS indicates real pathology, and in others it represents only a vigorous reactive change that is benign. In the United States, about 2.5 million ASCUS Pap results are reported each year. A survey of USA laboratories found that a median of 2.9% of all Pap smears are reported as ASCUS, with 10% of laboratories reporting more than 9% ASCUS results. Several strategies are currently in use to manage patients with ASCUS Pap smear results. Some clinicians repeat the Pap smear in 4 to 6 months. Many ASCUS patients directly undergo colposcopy to detect the 10 to 20% who prove to have an underlying higher-grade lesion, either LSIL or HSIL. Identifying women at high risk by testing for HPV avoids unnecessary colposcopy procedures. Patients with ASCUS who are positive for high-risk HPV are referred for colposcopy. Those who are negative for HPV undergo a repeat Pap smear at 6 months and 12 months. If these are also negative, the woman is returned to a routine screening schedule.

Colposcopy and biopsy are recommended for ASCUS Pap smears if the patient is positive for high-risk HPV types.

[Burd, E.M. (2003). Human papillomavirus and cervical cancer. *Clin Microbiol Rev. 2003 Jan; 16 (1): 1–17.* https://www.ncbi.nlm.nih.gov/pmc/articles/ PMC145302/]

Chapter 10
Self-Sampling for HPV

HPV self-sampling is an approach that could increase the testing frequency and be as effective as professional measures.

Self-sampling of vaginal cells is just as accurate as professionally-collected cervical cells for detecting severe dysplasia.

Dr. Caroline Hellsten at the Department of Obstetrics and Gynaecology of Lund University in Lund Sweden, and four medical colleagues, published an article in the July 2021 issue of the *European Journal of Cancer Prevention*. The study compared vaginal, self-sampled HPV tests with cervical, mid-wife-collected HPV tests. After studying over 28,000 women and examining the HPV-positive patients by follow-up Pap smears, severe dysplasia was detected in 0.48% of the self-sampled group and 0.47% of the cervical-sampled groups. Dr. Hellsten concluded:

> The self-sampling approach detects a similar proportion of severe dysplasia as regular screening. Thus, our study indicates that self-sampling could replace primary HPV screening of cervical samples.

[Hellsten, C., et al. (2021). Equal prevalence of severe cervical dysplasia by HPV self-sampling and by midwife-collected samples for primary HPV screening: a randomized controlled trial. *Eur J Cancer Prev. 2021 Jul 1; 30 (4): 334-340.* https://pubmed.ncbi.nlm.nih.gov/34010238/]

Moreover, self-sampled HPV tests appear to be equally effective as professionally-obtained cervical-sampled HPV tests to detect severe cervical dysplasia.

Self-sampling for HPV is convenient, widely accepted by patients and, most importantly, helps prevent cervical cancer deaths.

Dr. Ashwini Kamath Mulki at the Department of Family Medicine of Lehigh Valley Health Network in Allentown Pennsylvania, and a medical colleague, published an article in the January 2021 issue of the *BMC Women's Health* journal. Dr. Mulki evaluated self-sampling programs in various countries and said:

Screening for HPV has led to significant reductions in cervical cancer deaths in high-income countries. However, the same results have not been achieved in low- and middle-income countries. HPV self-sampling is a novel approach that could improve screening rates. This study's objective is to summarize the recent literature on HPV self-sampling. Fifty articles from 26 countries were included. Participation rates were very high in all studies, even when self-sampling was done at participants' homes, with over 89% participation. Overall, participants reported that HPV self-sampling was easy to perform, painless, and preferred over provider-collected sampling. The major benefits of self-sampling include convenience of screening from home, less embarrassment, and less travel. Improved education and awareness of self-sampling, combined with support from community health workers, could reduce perceptions of self-sampling being inferior to provider-collected sampling. Our literature review highlights that HPV self-sampling is a well-performing test that shows promise in terms of expanding screening efforts for the prevention of cervical cancer-related deaths.

[Mulki, A.K., et al. (2021). Human papillomavirus self-sampling performance in low- and middle-income countries. *BMC Women's Health. 2021 Jan 6; 21 (1): 12* https://pubmed.ncbi.nlm.nih.gov/33407355/]

These studies found that the acceptance of HPV self-sampling was positive. It was beneficial to enhance health awareness and promote cervical cancer screening frequency, especially among the under-screened populations.

HPV-negative tests do not rule out an HPV infection because (1) less than 10% of the known 228 HPV types are usually tested, and (2) the tests can yield false-negative results even for the few types tested. Therefore, treatment may be considered if HPV is suspected in the presence of HPV symptoms in the patient or the patient's partner.

Chapter 11
Degrees of Cervical Dysplasia

C ervical dysplasia is a condition in which cells of the cervix of the uterus become dysplastic or abnormal in appearance. In a small percentage of cases, dysplasia can develop into cancer, also called carcinoma in situ or invasive carcinoma. Dysplasia of the cervix of the uterus is usually detected first by an abnormal Pap smear.

CIN is an acronym for "Cervical Intraepithelial Neoplasia."

LGSIL (and LSIL) are acronyms for "Low-Grade Squamous Intraepithelial Lesion," such as CIN-1.

HGSIL (and HSIL) are acronyms for "High-Grade Squamous Intraepithelial Lesion," such as CIN-2 and CIN-3.

Depending on the laboratory terminology, the

lesions may be subdivided into degrees of dysplasia, such as mild, moderate, or severe. Some labs define the lesions as cervical intraepithelial neoplasias such as CIN-1, CIN-2, and CIN-3. Other labs will call them low-grade or high-grade squamous intraepithelial lesions, also known as LGSILs, or LSILs, and HGSILs, or HSILs.

LGSILs are mild dysplasia or low-grade lesions, also called CIN-1.

HGSILs are moderate-severe dysplasia or high-grade lesions, also called CIN-2 and CIN-3.

Dr. Michelle Khieu and Dr. Samantha L. Butler at the San Antonio Military Medical Center in San Antonio Texas published an article in the January 2022 issue of the *StatPearls* journal. Dr. Khieu said:

High-grade squamous intraepithelial lesion or HSIL encompasses the entities previously termed cervical intraepithelial neoplasia CIN-2, CIN-3, moderate and severe dysplasia and carcinoma in situ.

[Khieu, M., et al. (2022). High-grade squamous intraepithelial lesion. Treasure Island, Florida: *Stat-Pearls Publishing. January 5, 2022.* https://www.ncbi.nlm.nih.gov/books/NBK430728/]

It has been shown that one of the most critical factors of cancer potential is the presence of high-risk

HPV types. HPV typing provides the most rational basis for selecting women with LGSILs to be biopsied during colposcopy and treated or given follow-up with Pap smears.

Women with abnormal Pap smears may consider scheduling a colposcopy and biopsy for a better diagnosis, particularly if the HPV test is positive for high-risk HPV types.

Deeper involvement in the epithelial lining of the cervix earns the more severe labels such as CIN-2 and CIN-3, or severe dysplasia.

VIN is a variant that involves the vulva and is an acronym for "Vulvar Intraepithelial Neoplasia."

Other Paps may report ASCUS, the acronym for "Atypical Squamous Cells of Undetermined Significance," or AGUS, the acronym for "Atypical Glandular cells of Undetermined Significance."

Chapter 12
Colposcopy and Biopsy

C olposcopy is a procedure used as a diagnostic tool, not a screening tool. A scope and light are used to visualize the cervix under magnification using acetic acid 3% to highlight cervical lesions. At the same time, one or more biopsies may be taken from the surface of the cervix in the suspicious areas. If nothing looks suspicious, then biopsies may be taken blindly or randomly.

A biopsy refers to cutting away a piece of tissue with a surgical knife, usually the traditional biopsy forceps. This is standard for women with Pap smears indicating any grade of dysplasia and for women with repetitive Pap smears showing atypical squamous cells of undetermined significance (ASCUS).

Diagnostic accuracy for detecting cervical

dysplasia was 82.2% for Pap smears and 96.3% for colposcopy.

Dr. Fatemeh Sadat Najib at the Obstetrics and Gynecology Department of Shiraz University of Medical Sciences in Shiraz Iran, and five medical colleagues, published an article in the September 2020 issue of the *Indian Journal of Surgical Oncology*. Dr. Najib reported on the diagnostic accuracy of colposcopy in the detection of cervical lesions and said:

The overall diagnostic accuracy of the Pap smear and colposcopy was reported to be 82.2% and 96.3%, respectively. The results of this study demonstrate that colposcopy has a higher diagnostic accuracy in detecting cervical premalignant and malignant lesions compared to the Pap smear.

[Najib, F.S., et al. (2020). Diagnostic accuracy of cervical Pap smear and colposcopy in detecting premalignant and malignant lesions of cervix. *Indian J Surg Oncol. 2020 Sep; 11 (3): 453-458.* https://pubmed.ncbi.nlm.nih.gov/33013127/]

HPV testing combined with colposcopy was the most effective method for detecting CIN lesions.

Dr. Joanna Swiderska-Kiec at the Department of Obstetrics and Gynaecology of the Medical University of Warsaw in Warsaw Poland, and five medical colleagues, published an article in the May-June 2020 issue of the *In Vivo* journal comparing HPV testing with colposcopy. Dr. Swiderska-Kiec said:

> The aim of the study was to compare the diagnostic value of HPV testing and colposcopy in patients with abnormal cytology results. A total of 186 women with cytological abnormalities were included in the study. Combining HPV testing and colposcopy proved to be the most efficient method for detecting CIN lesions.

[Swiderska-Kiec, J., et al. (2020). Comparison of HPV testing and colposcopy in detecting cervical dysplasia in patients with cytological abnormalities. *In Vivo. May-Jun 2020; 34 (3): 1307-1315.* https://pubmed.ncbi.nlm.nih.gov/32354923/]

Moderate diagnostic accuracy was noted for colposcopy in patients who were HPV-positive and Pap smear-negative.

Dr. Yang Liu at the Department of Reproduction of Kunming Medical University in Kunming China, and seven medical colleagues, published an article in the March 2022 issue of the *Archives of Gynecology and Obstetrics* journal. The article concerned the diagnostic value of colposcopy in HPV-positive patients with negative Pap smears. It concluded that the Pap smear false-negative rate was 43.2% and that colposcopy was more accurate in patients with HPV 16 or 18, which are HR, or high-risk, types. Dr. Liu found that colposcopy in HPV-positive, Pap smear-negative patients has a moderate diagnostic accuracy.

[Liu, Y., et al. (2022). Diagnostic value of colposcopy in patients with cytology-negative and HR-HPV-positive cervical lesions. *Arch Gynecol Obstet. 2022 Mar 23.* https://pubmed.ncbi.nlm.nih.gov/35320389/]

A colposcopy allows for a closer look than a Pap smear does. A colposcopy may include random or directed needle-type biopsies, especially when a lesion can be seen. The conclusion is this: a colposcopy is better at diagnosing and evaluating visible dysplasia, but a Pap smear is better for screening mild dysplasia with no visible lesion.

Chapter 13
HPV Tests and False-Negative Results

An HPV test typically requires a swab of the cervix, anus, penile urethra, or oral cavity. It can also be performed on a biopsy of a wart, the cervix, or the vagina. An Ob-Gyn doctor generally performs it for women, and a urologist performs it for men.

Most HPV tests detect only a few HPV types representing the most common or serious types. These types may be divided into three groups: low-risk, moderate-risk, and high-risk.

The HPV test determines in which groups the detected HPV types reside. Some HPV tests determine a few specific types, such as HPV 16 and 18, plus another 12-14 high-risk types as a group. Other HPV tests may determine just a single group of 14 high-risk types.

HPV-negative tests do not rule out an HPV infection because (1) less than 10% of the known 228 HPV types are usually tested, and (2) the tests can yield false-negative results even for the few types tested. Therefore, treatment may be considered if HPV is suspected in the presence of HPV symptoms in the patient or the patient's partner.

Dr. D.A.M. Heideman at the Department of Pathology of VU University Medical Center in Amsterdam Netherlands, and eight medical colleagues, published an article in the November 2013 issue of the *Journal of Clinical Microbiology.* Dr. Heideman said: "The Aptima HPV assay is an FDA-approved assay for detecting human papillomavirus from 14 high-risk HPV types (16, 18, 31, 33, 35, 39, 45, 51, 52, 56, 58, 59, 66, and 68)."

[Heideman, D.A.M., et al. (2013). The Aptima HPV assay fulfills the cross-sectional clinical and repro-ducibility criteria of international guidelines for human papillomavirus test requirements for cervical screening. *J Clin Microbiol. 2013 Nov; 51 (11): 3653–3657.* https://www.ncbi.nlm.nih.gov/pmc/articles/PMC3889747/]

Dr. Maio Cui and seven medical colleagues at the Department of Pathology of Mount Sinai School of Medicine in New York New York published an article in the June 2014 issue of the *Journal of Clinical Microbiology* about the Roche Cobas 4800 HPV test. Dr. Cui said: "The Roche Cobas 4800 HPV test can detect HPV-16, HPV-18, and 12 other high-risk HPVs (31, 33, 35, 39, 45, 51, 52, 56, 58, 59, 66, and 68) as a pooled result."

[Cui, M., et al. (2014). Clinical performance of Roche Cobas 4800 HPV test. *J Clin Microbiol. 2014 Jun; 52 (6):* 2210–2211. https://www.ncbi.nlm.nih.gov/pmc/articles/ PMC4042746/]

The HPV test may be false-negative, meaning it fails to detect HPV even when HPV is present. This is obviously true for the 90% of HPV types that the HPV test was not designed to detect.

HPV tests may produce false-negative results *even for specific types they are designed to detect.*

Dr. Hana Jaworek at the Institute of Molecular and Translational Medicine of Palacky University in Olomouc Czech Republic, and five medical colleagues, published an article in the August 2019 issue of the *Public Library of Science* journal about false-negative HPV tests. Dr. Jaworek said:

HPV 68 is a probable carcinogenic HPV genotype which is included in almost all HPV screening assays and exists as two genetically variable subtypes: HPV

68a and HPV 68b. Routine HPV sample testing has shown that the Cobas 4800 HPV Test by Roche provides higher false-negative rates for HPV 68 status than PapilloCheck HPV-Screening by Greiner Bio-One. The HPV 68a subtype was missed by Cobas 4800 in more than 85% of all HPV 68a-positive cases. Therefore, commercially available assays may underestimate HPV 68 prevalence.

[Jaworek, H., et al. (2019). Pitfalls of commercially available HPV tests in HPV 68a detection. *PLoS One. 2019 Aug 5; 14 (8): e0220373.* https://pubmed.ncbi.nlm. nih.gov/31381580/]

Dr. Anna Macios at the Centre of Postgraduate Medical Education in Warsaw Poland and a medical colleague published an article in the June 2022 issue of the *Diagnostics Basel* journal. Dr. Macios said:

False-negative results in cervical cancer screening pose serious risks to women. We present a comprehensive literature review on the risks and reasons of obtaining the false negative results of primary cervical cancer screening tests and discuss their clinical and public health impact. For high-risk human papillomavirus molecular tests, those include truly non-HPV-associated tumors, lesions driven by low-risk HPV types, and clearance of HPV genetic material before sampling.

[Macios, A., et al. (2022). False-negative results in cervical cancer screening - risks, reasons, and implications for clinical practice and public health. *Diagnostics (Basel). 2022 Jun 20; 12 (6): 1508.* https://pubmcd.ncbi. nlm.nih.gov/35741319/]

Dr. Mario Poljak at the Faculty of Medicine of the University of Ljubljana in Ljubljana Slovenia, and four medical colleagues, published an article in the September 2020 issue of the *Clinical Microbiology and Infection* journal. They discussed the available HPV tests. Dr. Poljak said:

We identified 254 distinct commercial HPV tests. 60% of the HPV tests on the global market are still without a single peer-reviewed publication. Furthermore, 82% of tests lack any published analytical and/or clinical evaluation, and over 90% are not evaluated in line with consensus requirements that ensure safe use in clinical settings. Significant challenges and scope for improvement still exist for both the HPV scientific community and the manufacturers of HPV tests. The latter must put more effort into validating their products.

[Poljak, M., et al. (2020). Commercially available molecular tests for human papillomaviruses: a global overview. *Clin Microbiol Infect. 2020 Sep; 26 (9): 1144-1150.* https://pubmed.ncbi.nlm.nih.gov/32247892/]

- does test have peer reviewed publication?
- published, analytical/clinical evaluation

Part III: Transmission and Prevalence of HPV

Chapter 14
HPV Transmission in General

Some HPV types are primarily transmitted sexually but can also be transmitted through methods such as a handshake, manicure, haircut, waxing, or other salon procedure. Any skin-to-skin contact may transmit HPV as suggested by the prevalence of antibodies to certain HPV types, including high-risk, even among school children.

Transmission of HPV via floor or seat surfaces is highly unlikely.

Dr. Mirja Puranen and two medical colleagues at the Department of Pathology of the University of Kuopio in Finland published an article in the 1996 issue of the *Scandinavian Journal of Infectious Diseases*. Dr. Puranen explained:

To evaluate the transmission of genital human papillomavirus through the floor and seats of humid dwellings, samples were collected with a toothbrush from the floor and seat surfaces of humid dwellings; showers, saunas, and dressing rooms. No HPV DNA-positive samples were found. These results indicate that transmission of genital HPV infection via floor or seat surfaces in the above dwellings in general or family use is highly unlikely.

[Puranen, M., et al. (1996). Transmission of genital human papillomavirus infections is unlikely through the floor and seats of humid dwellings in countries of high-level hygiene. *Scand J Infect Dis. 1996; 28 (3): 243-6.* https://pubmed.ncbi.nlm.nih.gov/8863354/]

HPV was detected on the fingertips of men and women with genital warts suggesting that any skin-to-skin contact can result in the transmission of the virus.

Dr. C. Sonnex and two medical colleagues at the Department of GU Medicine of Addenbrooke's Hospital in Cambridge England published an article in the October 1999 issue of the journal of *Sexually Transmitted Infections*. The article revealed that HPV was detected on the fingers of patients with genital warts. Dr. Sonnex examined 14 men and 8 women with genital warts who had brush samples taken from genital lesions, finger-tips, and tips of fingernails. HPV was detected in all 8 female genital samples and 13 male genital samples. HPV was seen in the finger brush samples of 3 women and 9 men. Dr. Sonnex said:

> This study has identified hand carriage of genital HPV types in patients with genital warts. Although sexual intercourse is considered the usual mode of transmitting genital HPV infection, our findings raise the possibility of transmission by finger-genital contact.

[Sonnex, C., et al. (1999). Detection of human papillomavirus DNA on the fingers of patients with genital warts. *Sex Transm Infect. 1999 Oct; 75 (5): 317-9.* https://pubmed.ncbi.nlm.nih.gov/10616355/]

First-time HPV infection developed in 32.3% of female university students within 24 months, and condoms were not protective.

Dr. Rachel L. Winer and five medical colleagues at the Department of Epidemiology of the University of Washington in Seattle Washington published an article in the February 2003 issue of the *American Journal of Epidemiology*. These doctors followed 603 female university students for two years. At 4-month intervals, cervical and vaginal samples were collected to detect

HPV. At 24 months, the cumulative incidence of first-time infection was 32.3%. Dr. Winer concluded:

> Always using male condoms with a new partner was not protective. Infection in virgins was rare, but any type of nonpenetrative sexual contact was associated with an increased risk. Detection of oral HPV was rare and was not associated with oral-penile contact. The data show that the incidence of HPV associated with acquisition of a new sex partner is high.

[Winer, R.L., et al. (2003). Genital human papillomavirus infection: incidence and risk factors in a cohort of female university students. *Am J Epidemiol. 2003 Feb 1; 157 (3): 218-26.* https://pubmed.ncbi.nlm.nih.gov/12543621/]

Antibodies to HPV 1 and 2 were found in 37.5-51.9% of 11-13 year-old school girls. Antibodies to high-risk HPV 16 were found in 7.6%.

Dr. H.A. Cubie and five medical colleagues at the Regional Clinical Virology Laboratory of City Hospital in Edinburgh Scotland published an article in the November 1998 issue of the *Journal of Medical Virology*. Dr. Cubie found HPV antibodies in 11-13 year-old school girls. Antibodies to HPV 2 were detected in 37.5%, and antibodies to HPV 1 were detected in 51.9%. Dr. Cubie said: "Antibodies to both HPV 1 and HPV 2 were found frequently, being present in 29.7%."

[Cubie, H.A., et al. (1998). Presence of antibodies to human papillomavirus virus-like particles (VLPs) in 11-13-year-old schoolgirls. *J Med Virol. 1998 Nov; 56 (3): 210-6.* https://pubmed.ncbi.nlm.nih.gov/9783687/]

HPV was detected in 36% of pubic hair samples and 50% of perianal hair samples of patients with genital warts.

Dr. Ingeborg L. A. Boxman and four medical colleagues at the Department of Virology Academic Medical Center in Amsterdam Netherlands published an article in the July 1999 issue of the *Journal of Clinical Microbiology.* They detected HPV 6 and 11 in pubic hair and perianal hair from patients with genital warts. HPV was detected in 36% of pubic hair samples and 50% of perianal hair samples.

[Boxman, I.L.A., et al. (1999). Detection of human papillomavirus types 6 and 11 in pubic and perianal hair from patients with genital warts. *J Clin Microbiol. 1999 Jul; 37 (7): 2270-3.* https://pubmed.ncbi.nlm.nih.gov/10364596/]

Based on these studies, the transmission of HPV non-sexually is not only possible but quite common.

Chapter 15
HPV Transmission during Childbirth

Transmission of HPV is common at the time of delivery, but serious infection in the newborn is rare.

Transmission of HPV during childbirth may occur in 80% of deliveries by infected women.

Dr. Patrizia Tenti and five medical colleagues at the Department of Human Pathology of the University of Pavia in Pavia Italy published an article in the April 1999 issue of the *Obstetrics and Gynecology* journal on the transmission of HPV during childbirth. According to Dr. Tenti, the study consisted of 711 pregnant women. Newborns were HPV-negative in which membranes ruptured less than 2 hours before delivery. When rupture preceded delivery by 2-4 hours, and when it occurred after more than 4 hours, the rates for HPV positivity in newborns were 33% and 80%, respectively. Even so, at follow-up, the HPV virus was cleared from the newborn oral samples as early as the 5th week after delivery. Dr. Tenti said:

> Pregnant women with latent HPV infections have low potential of transmitting the virus to the oropharyngeal mucosae of their infants. The time between rupture of the amnion and delivery seems to be a critical factor in predicting transmission. Human papillomavirus–positive infants should be considered contaminated rather than infected since the virus is cleared over several months after birth.

[Tenti, P., et al. (1999). Perinatal transmission of human papillomavirus from gravidas with latent infections. *Obstet Gynecol. 1999 Apr; 93 (4): 475-9.* https://pubmed.ncbi.nlm.nih.gov/10214817/]

HPV transmission occurs from at least 30% of HPV-positive mothers to their infants.

Dr. Phillip S. Rice and three medical colleagues at the Department of Virology of Saint Thomas's Medical School in London England published an article in the January 1999 issue of the *Reviews of Medical Virology* journal. They presented evidence of HPV transmission from HPV-positive mothers to their infants. Dr. Rice states:

> We present evidence for vertical transmission from at least 30% of HPV-positive mothers to their infants, resulting in persistent infection in children. That the mother is the source of infant infection has been confirmed by DNA sequencing. We also discuss the evidence for oral HPV-16 infection in children. In our own studies, HPV-16 DNA was detected in buccal cells from 48% of children, aged 3-11, and active infection was confirmed in some children. Other studies have reported prevalences of 19-27% among children less than 11 years of age. Serological studies also suggest that up to 45% of prepubertal children have acquired HPV-16. Thus, convincing evidence is now available for vertical transmission of high-risk HPVs, which probably results in widespread infection among children.

[Rice, P.S., et al. (1999). High-risk genital papillomavirus infections are spread vertically. *Rev Med Virol.* *Jan-Mar 1999; 9 (1): 15-21.* https://pubmed.ncbi.nlm.nih.gov/10371668/]

Treatment of HPV infection during pregnancy is

recommended to avoid transmission during childbirth.

Dr. Mihaela C. Radu at the Obstetrics and Gynecology Hospital in Ploiesti Romania, and eight medical colleagues, published an article in the June 2021 issue of the *Cureus Journal of Medical Science*. Dr. Radu reported on findings about HPV at the time of childbirth and believes that HPV infection during pregnancy must be treated to avoid transmitting it to the newborn baby. Dr. Radu said: "We believe that HPV infection during pregnancy must be treated when detected in order to avoid transmitting it to the newborn baby."

[Radu, M.C., et al. (2021). Human papillomavirus infection at the time of delivery. *Cureus. 2021 Jun 1; 13 (6): e15364.* https://pubmed.ncbi.nlm.nih.gov/ 34094788/]

Although severe infection is rare in infants exposed to HPV during childbirth, some recommend treatment during pregnancy. A cesarean section may also be considered when HPV is present at the time of delivery.

Chapter 16
Cervical Dysplasia during Pregnancy

C ervical dysplasia appears to be more common during pregnancy, but the main reason is that Pap smears are standard protocol during a routine pregnancy exam. Obviously with more tests more detection will occur.

Another reason for more detection during pregnancy is that a woman's immune system is stressed during this time. This immune system stress makes it easier for the HPV virus to evade the immune system and damage cervical cells.

Cervical dysplasia present during pregnancy will after delivery regress in 10-70% and progress in 3-30% of cases.

Dr. Antonio Frega and eight medical colleagues at the Department of Gynecology of Sapienza University in Rome Italy published an article in the July-August 2007 issue of the journal of *Anticancer Research*. They studied cervical dysplasia during pregnancy and in the postpartum period. Dr. Frega reported:

> Of dysplasia cases diagnosed during pregnancy, 10-70% regress and sometimes even disappear postpartum, while persistence in the severity of cervical neoplasia is reported in 25-47% and progression occurs in 3-30%.

[Frega, A., et al. (2007). Clinical management and follow-up of squamous intraepithelial cervical lesions during pregnancy and postpartum. *Anticancer Res. Jul-Aug 2007; 27 (4C): 2743-6*. https://pubmed.ncbi.nlm.nih.gov/17695441/]

Cervical dysplasia during pregnancy is not a risk for pre-term delivery or pre-eclampsia complications.

Dr. Taliya Lantsman at the Department of Obstetrics and Gynecology of Feinberg School of Medicine of Northwestern University in Chicago Illinois, and seven medical colleagues, published an article in the July 2020 issue of the *American Journal of Perinatology*. They reviewed the association of cervical dysplasia during pregnancy to evaluate any adverse events such as preterm delivery or pre-eclampsia. After studying 2,814 women, cervical dysplasia during pregnancy was not associated with these particular complications.

[Lantsman, T., et al. (2020). Association between cervical dysplasia and adverse pregnancy outcomes. *Am J Perinatol. 2020 Jul; 37 (9): 947-954.* https://pubmed. ncbi.nlm.nih.gov/31167238/]

In light of the studies mentioned above, cervical dysplasia does not appear to constitute any particular risk *per se* during pregnancy other than the possible transmission of HPV during childbirth and miscarriages during early pregnancy.

Chapter 17
Prevalence and Public Awareness of HPV

The prevalence of HPV is high, but awareness of it is low, not only in the general public but also in the medical community.

Over 42 million persons - 13% of the population - are currently infected with HPV in the USA, with 13 million new cases annually.

These estimates are probably low since they are based on HPV testing. HPV-negative tests do not rule out an HPV infection because (1) less than 10% of the known 228 HPV types are usually tested, and (2) the tests can yield false-negative results even for the few types tested.

Dr. Rayleen M. Lewis at the Centre de Recherche of the Université Laval in Quebec Canada, and seven medical colleagues, published an article in the April

2021 issue of the journal of *Sexually Transmitted Diseases*. The article discussed the prevalence of HPV infections. Dr. Lewis found:

An estimated 23.4 million men and 19.2 million women had a disease-associated HPV type infection in 2018. We document a high HPV burden of infection in the United States in 2018, with 42 million persons infected with disease-associated HPV and 13 million persons acquiring a new infection. Although most infections clear, some disease-associated HPV type infections progress to disease.

[Lewis, R.M., et al. (2021). Estimated prevalence and incidence of disease-associated human papillomavirus types among 15-59 year-olds in the United States. *Sex Transm Dis. 2021 Apr 1; 48 (4): 273-277.* https://pubmed.ncbi.nlm.nih.gov/33492097/]

Approximately 80% of women will acquire an HPV infection by age 50.

Dr. Kari P. Braaten and a medical colleague at the Division of Gynecology of Children's Hospital in Boston Massachusetts published an article in the Winter 2008 issue of the *Reviews in Obstetrics and Gynecology* journal. Dr. Braaten said: "Human papillomavirus is the most common sexually transmitted infection in the United

States with approximately 80% of women having acquired an infection by the age of 50."

[Braaten, K.P., et al. (2008). Human Papillomavirus (HPV), HPV-Related Disease, and the HPV Vaccine. *Rev Obstet Gynecol. 2008 Winter; 1 (1): 2–10.* https://www.ncbi.nlm.nih.gov/pmc/articles/PMC2492590/]

Less than half of the women undergoing genital warts treatment knew that HPV causes cancer, is sexually transmitted, is common, and often goes away on its own without treatment.

Dr. Jill Koshiol at the National Cancer Institute of the National Institutes of Health in Bethesda Maryland, and three medical colleagues, published an article in the June 2009 issue of the *Journal of Health Communication.* They discussed the general public's knowledge about HPV. Specifically, the study aimed to evaluate knowledge about HPV in women with genital warts compared to women without genital warts. Dr. Koshiol said:

> Women who reported treatment for genital warts were more likely to have heard of HPV, to have been told they had HPV, and to have accurate information about HPV, such as that HPV causes cancer. However, a large proportion of women who reported treatment for genital warts had not heard of HPV.

Dr. Koshiol also noted:

Fifty-eight percent of women reporting treatment for genital warts and 38% of women reporting no treatment for genital warts had heard of HPV. Of the women reporting treatment for genital warts, 41% had never heard of or were unsure if they had heard of HPV. Less than half of the women reporting genital warts treatment who had heard of HPV also reported being told that they had HPV. Similarly, less than half of the women reporting genital warts treatment knew that HPV causes cancer, is sexually transmitted, is common, and often goes away on its own without treatment. Of those women asked about HPV and pregnancy, the most common response was that HPV did affect their ability to get pregnant, regardless of genital warts status.

More concerning was the limited knowledge of health care providers about HPV. This may explain why the patients seem to lack accurate information.

Only 29% of Family Physicians and 67% of Ob-Gyn specialists knew that HPV could clear without medical intervention.

Dr. Koshiol points out:

Two recent surveys of USA clinicians found that only 33-40% overall knew that HPV could clear without medical intervention, although Obstetrician-Gynecologists were much more likely to know that HPV clears spontaneously than physicians in Family or Internal Medicine, 67% versus 35% and 29%, respectively. While these studies found that nearly all physicians knew that persistent HPV infection increases the risk of cervical dysplasia and cancer, a survey of 2,748 members of the American Academy of Family Physicians found that only 20% listed HPV as a risk factor for cervical cancer. Further, many clinicians are unaware that the HPV types that cause genital warts differ from those that cause cervical cancer.

[Koshiol, J., et al. (2009). Knowledge of human papillomavirus. *J Health Commun. 2009 Jun; 14 (4): 331–345.* https://www.ncbi.nlm.nih.gov/pmc/articles/PMC2768561/]

It is not surprising that patients often lack basic medical knowledge about HPV. But, remarkably, only 67% of Ob-Gyn specialists and only 29% of Family Physicians know that HPV can clear spontaneously.

Part IV: Treatment of Cervical Dysplasia

Chapter 18
Medical Treatments for Cervical Dysplasia

T he most common medical therapies for cervical dysplasia include TCA, also known as trichloroacetic acid, and 5-FU, also known as 5-fluorouracil or Efudex® cream. 5-FU and TCA appear to be of little benefit in some studies; however, in at least one study, patients treated with 5-FU performed twice as well as the control group.

Trichloroacetic acid and 5-fluorouracil cream had no beneficial effect on cervical dysplasia in a study of 77 women.

Dr. N. Husseinzadeh and two medical colleagues at the Department of Obstetrics and Gynecology of the University of Cincinnati College of Medicine in Cincinnati Ohio published an article in the October 1994 issue of *The Journal of Reproductive Medicine* about treatment outcomes for HPV and cervical dysplasia. These doctors explained that 77 women with HPV changes associated with cervical dysplasia were studied. All were treated with the laser for cervical lesions and with either 5-fluorouracil cream or trichloroacetic acid. There was no significant difference between those who had no treatment and those who received 5-FU or TCA. Dr. Husseinzadeh said: "It appears that the treatment modalities used in this study did not have any beneficial effect on associated subclinical HPV infections."

[Husseinzadeh, N., et al. (1994). Subclinical cervicovaginal human papillomavirus infections associated with cervical condylomata and dysplasia. Treatment outcomes. *The Journal of Reproductive Medicine, 01 Oct 1994, 39 (10): 777-780.* https://pubmed.ncbi.nlm.nih.gov/7837123/]

Treatment with 5-FU cream for cervical dysplasia had 50% success at six months in one study of 60 women.

Dr. Lisa Rahangdale at the Department of Obstetrics and Gynecology of the University of North Carolina School of Medicine in Chapel Hill North Carolina, and five medical colleagues, published an article in the April 2014 issue of the *American Journal of Obstetrics and Gynecology* about the topical use of 5-FU for cervical dysplasia. Dr. Rahangdale reported that women in the

5-FU group were treated with intra-vaginal 5-FU once every two weeks for a total of 4 months. At the 6-month evaluation, 50% of the 5-FU group had a documented normal biopsy, normal Pap smear, and negative HPV test compared with only 22% in the control group. Dr. Rahangdale concluded:

> Topical 5-FU appears to be an effective medical therapy for CIN-2 in young women. 5-FU is readily available and may be considered as an off-label treatment option for young women with CIN-2 who are interested in the treatment of disease but want to avoid excisional procedures.

[Rahangdale, L., et al. (2014). Topical 5-fluorouracil for treatment of cervical intraepithelial neoplasia 2: a randomized controlled trial. *Am J Obstet Gynecol. 2014 Apr; 210 (4): 314.e1-314.e8.* https://pubmed.ncbi.nlm.nih.gov/24384495/]

Studies of some medical treatments for cervical dysplasia have shown that 5-FU is more effective than TCA and appears slightly better than the results expected in untreated individuals based on the natural history of the disease.

Chapter 19
Surgical Treatments for
Cervical Dysplasia

The most common surgical therapies for cervical dysplasia include LEEP, CKC, and cryotherapy or freezing.

LEEP is an acronym for "**L**oop **E**lectrosurgical **E**xcision **P**rocedure."

CKC is an acronym for "**C**old **K**nife **C**one."

A LEEP and a CKC refer to types of conizations or cone biopsies for treating cervical dysplasia. A cone biopsy can be done with a knife or scalpel, called a cold knife cone. Usually, the term "cone biopsy" refers to a cold knife cone. But a cone biopsy can also be done with a laser or an electrosurgical instrument referred to as a LEEP.

[Cooper, D.B., et al. (2021). Conization of cervix. Treasure Island, Florida: *StatPearls Publishing. December*

2021. https://www.ncbi.nlm.nih.gov/books/ NBK441845/]

LEEP procedures are usually performed with one of three loop sizes. There is less risk of surgical complications if the smaller loops will suffice to remove the dysplasia. In addition, the increased experience of the doctor can decrease the risk of surgical complications. Perhaps the most frequent issue is simply a failure to cure the problem, and the risk of complications increases with each additional surgery.

After a LEEP procedure, 27.5% had recurrent cervical dysplasia during the next five years, indicating a 72.5% success.

Dr. C.A. Livasy and three medical colleagues at the Department of Pathology and Laboratory Medicine of the University of North Carolina in Chapel Hill North Carolina published an article in the March 1999 issue of the *Modern Pathology* journal. It concerned predictors of recurrent cervical dysplasia following a LEEP procedure. They studied 248 patients with CIN-3 treated by LEEP over five years. Fifty-five patients, or 27.5%, had recurrent dysplasia.

[Livasy, C.A., et al. (1999). Predictors of recurrent dysplasia after a cervical loop electrocautery excision procedure for CIN-3: a study of margin, endocervical gland, and quadrant involvement. *Mod Pathol. 1999*

Mar; 12 (3): 233-8. https://pubmed.ncbi.nlm.nih.gov/10102607/]

When the results of this study are compared to the natural history of the disease over five years, LEEP did not have a significant benefit. The untreated natural history of cervical dysplasia yields approximately the same percentage of success.

After a cone biopsy, antibodies and immunity to HPV developed by 27 months in 82% of the women.

Dr. Kristina Elfgren and five medical colleagues at the Department of Obstetrics and Gynecology of Huddinge University Hospital in Stockholm Sweden published an article in the March 1996 issue of the *American Journal of Obstetrics and Gynecology.* They studied the value of cervical conization for cervical dysplasia. Dr. Elfgren measured antibodies against HPV to determine the immune response resulting from the surgical procedure of a cone biopsy. The results were encouraging since 19 of 23 women, or 82%, were disease-free after 27 months. Dr. Elfgren concluded:

> Human papillomavirus was regularly eliminated, and human papillomavirus antibody levels declined after efficient treatment, suggesting that conization may be effective for treating the underlying human papillomavirus infection.

This study's main point is that most patients developed immunity following the cone biopsy; however, the success statistics for cone biopsy are similar to those for women who received no treatment at all, even though the success was slightly better than for the LEEP.

[Elfgren, K., et al. (1996). Conization for cervical intraepithelial neoplasia is followed by the disappearance of human papillomavirus deoxyribonucleic acid and a decline in serum and cervical mucus antibodies against human papillomavirus antigens. *Am J Obstet Gynecol. 1996 Mar; 174 (3): 937-42.* https://pubmed.ncbi.nlm.nih.gov/8633673/]

Cervical excisional surgeries for cervical dysplasia increase the risk of spontaneous preterm birth, premature rupture of membranes, chorioamnionitis, low birth weight infants, admission to neonatal intensive care, and perinatal mortality.

Dr. M. Kyrgiou at the Institute of Reproductive and Developmental Biology of the Faculty of Medicine of Imperial College in London England, and eight medical colleagues, published an article in the July 2016 issue of the *British Medical Journal*. They evaluated the risk of complications after surgical treatment for cervical dysplasia in 71 studies. Dr. Kyrgiou said:

Treatment significantly increased the risk. Compared with no treatment, the risk of preterm birth was higher in women who had undergone more than one treatment and with increasing cone depth. Spontaneous preterm birth, premature rupture of the membranes, chorioamnionitis, low birth weight, admission to neonatal intensive care, and perinatal mortality were also significantly increased after treatment. The frequency and severity of adverse sequelae increase with increasing cone depth.

[Kyrgiou, M., et al. (2016). Adverse obstetric outcomes after local treatment for cervical pre-invasive and early invasive disease according to cone depth: systematic review and meta-analysis. *BMJ. 2016; 354: i3633.* https://pubmed.ncbi.nlm.nih.gov/27469988/]

Dr. Marco Monti at the Department of Maternal and Child Health and Urological Sciences of Sapienza University in Rome Italy, and twelve medical colleagues, published an article in the April 2021 issue of the journal of *Minerva Obstetrics and Gynecology.* They compared cervical surgeries for dysplasia with obstetrical complications of preterm delivery, low birth weight infants, and premature membrane rupture. Surgeries evaluated included loop electrosurgical excision procedure, large loop excision of the transformation zone, cold-knife conization, and laser conization. All surgeries showed an increased risk of preterm delivery, low birth weight infants, and premature rupture of membranes, especially for the large loop excision of the transformation zone proce-dure and the cold-knife conization surgery. Dr. Monti said:"Moreover, the increase of preterm delivery was associated with cone size, cervical length, repeated treatment and a short conization-to-pregnancy interval."

[Monti, M., et al. (2021). Relationship between cervical excisional treatment for cervical intraepithelial neoplasia and obstetrical outcome. *Minerva Obstet Gynecol. 2021 Apr; 73 (2): 233-246.* https://pubmed.ncbi. nlm.nih.gov/33140628/]

Cone biopsy with cold knife cone appears to have more complications than LEEP. Still, both procedures have some success in stimulating immunity similar to the natural history of the disease.

LEEP and cone biopsy complications are relatively rare but can be severe. Your doctor will usually suggest that you postpone pregnancy for at least one year after a LEEP or cone biopsy so that the cervix can fully heal from the surgery. Cervical incompetence can make it challenging to carry pregnancies to term. This some-times results in miscarriages or preterm delivery because the cervix is too thin to keep the uterus closed during the later stages of pregnancy.

Infection can occur following a LEEP or cone biopsy. Pelvic discomfort during the procedure and cramping afterward are both common.

Stenosis, or shrinking of the cervical canal, can occur due to scarring. It is the most frequent LEEP complication, occurring in 4.3% of cases. However, stenosis is more common with a cone biopsy because a cone biopsy does not allow for good control of the incision depth and angle. A cone biopsy may remove more tissue than a LEEP and is generally used when dysplasia in the cervical canal is suspected of going beyond the reach of the LEEP.

Cervical stenosis occurs in 4.3% of LEEP procedures and 10.2% of laser conizations.

Dr. J.J. Baldauf and five medical colleagues at Service de Gynecologie Obstetrique of Hopitaux Universitaires in Strasbourg France published an article in 1997 in the *Journal of Gynecology, Obstetrics and Biology Reproduction*. Dr. Baldauf reported on the consequences of cervical stenosis and said: "Stenosis complicated 10.2% of the laser conizations and 4.3% of the LEEPs."

[Baldauf, J.J., et al. (1997). Consequences and treatment of cervical stenoses after laser conization or loop electrosurgical excision. *J Gynecol Obstet Biol Reprod (Paris). 1997; 26 (1): 64-70.* https://pubmed.ncbi.nlm.nih.gov/9091546/]

Unfortunately, some women may endure surgery several times until the dysplasia is gone. Even a hysterectomy may not cure the problem. Some women will continue to have abnormal Paps and dysplasia in the vaginal wall following a hysterectomy because a hysterectomy may not stimulate immunity to eliminate the HPV infection.

Ideally some of the cells harboring the HPV virus may be disrupted during surgery, thus allowing the immune cells to engage the HPV virus.

Cervical epithelial cells are called poor APCs, an acronym for "**A**ntigen-**P**resenting **C**ells," because they do not effectively present the HPV antigen to the immune cells. If the immune cells can identify the HPV virus, they can respond appropriately and develop an immune response. This immune response is probably why all these surgical procedures work to some degree, and one is not significantly more successful than the other. It might be more effective if the surgeon simply used a fine wire brush and scraped up the cervix, thus disrupting the cervical epithelial cells and thereby exposing the HPV virus to the immune cells.

Cryosurgery treatment for cervical dysplasia had no adverse effect on the onset of labor or the infant.

Dr. Erik Hemmingsson at the Department of Gynaecological Oncology of University Hospital in Uppsala Sweden published an article in the August 1982 issue of the *British Journal of Obstetrics and Gynecology.* He studied the outcome of third-trimester pregnancies after cryotherapy of the cervix. Dr. Hemmingsson said:

> It was concluded that cryosurgery of the cervix had no effect on the onset or progress of labour, or on the infant, an important advantage compared with cold-knife conization as a therapy for young women with cervical intraepithelial neoplasia.

[Hemmingsson, E. (1982). Outcome of third-trimester pregnancies after cryotherapy of the uterine cervix. *Br J Obstet Gynaecol. 1982 Aug; 89 (8): 675-7.* https://pubmed.ncbi.nlm.nih.gov/7104260/]

Some doctors prefer cryotherapy to other surgical methods for cervical dysplasia because it does not cause cervical incompetence. Following cryotherapy, most doctors advise patients to avoid sex for 4-6 weeks, when patients may experience a watery-bloody discharge.

A comparison of LEEP and cryotherapy shows

each has slight advantages and disadvantages over the other.

Dr. Pietro D'Alessandro at the Department of Neuroscience School of Medicine of the University of Naples in Naples Italy, and six medical colleagues, published an article in the October 2018 issue of the journal of *Gynecology and Minimally Invasive Therapy.* They compared the effectiveness of LEEP to cryotherapy for cervical dysplasia. Dr. D'Alessandro said:

> In women with CIN, treatment with LEEP was associated with a significantly lower risk of persistence of disease at 6 months and recurrence of disease at 12 months compared to treatment with cryotherapy.

[D'Alessandro, P., et al. (2018). Loop electrosurgical excision procedure versus cryotherapy in the treatment of cervical intraepithelial neoplasia: A systematic review and meta-analysis of randomized controlled trials. *Gynecol Minim Invasive Ther. 2018 Oct-Dec; 7 (4): 145–151.* https://pubmed.ncbi.nlm.nih.gov/30306032/]

In summary, LEEP surgery has 72.5% success over five years with the complication of cervical stenosis in 4.3%, whereas cone biopsy has 82% success at 27 months with the complication of cervical stenosis in

10.2%. Both procedures have the risk of pre-term delivery due to cervical incompetence.

If surgery is chosen, cryosurgery may be preferable since less damage is done to the cervix. However, the persistence or recurrence of cervical dysplasia is greater with cryosurgery than with a LEEP.

Chapter 20
Beta-Carotene, Folic Acid, and Vitamin C Treatment for Cervical Dysplasia

S ome speculation is that the use of beta-carotene, folic acid, and vitamin C may influence the course of cervical dysplasia. This may be true in some cases, but the effect does not seem significant based on the following studies.

Vitamin C and beta-carotene did not significantly influence the natural history of cervical dysplasia over two years.

Dr. D. Mackerras and seven medical colleagues at the Department of Public Health and Community Medicine of the University of Sydney in Sydney Australia published an article in the March 1999 issue of the *British Journal of Cancer*. Dr. Mackerras found that beta-carotene and vitamin C, when taken by 141 women with minor cervical dysplasia, did not have a significant influence on the natural history of cervical dysplasia over two years. 43 lesions regressed to normal, and 13 progressed to CIN-2. Dr. Mackerras said:

> The currently available evidence from this and other trials suggests that high doses of these compounds are unlikely to increase the regression or decrease the progression of minor atypia and CIN I.

[Mackerras, D., et al. (1999). Randomized double-blind trial of beta-carotene and vitamin C in women with minor cervical abnormalities. *Br J Cancer. 1999 Mar; 79 (9-10): 1448–1453.* https://pubmed.ncbi.nlm.nih.gov/10188889/]

Folic acid and beta-carotene did not help prevent cervical cancer.

Dr. Anna R. Giliano of the Arizona Prevention Center at the University of Arizona in Tucson Arizona published an article in the January 1998 issue of the *Nutrition Review* journal. She studied the use of folic acid and beta-carotene but found that there was no particular benefit for the prevention of cervical cancer. Dr. Giliano said:

> Research from the last two decades suggests a role for nutrients in the prevention of cervical cancer.

However, results from phase III folic acid and β-carotene chemo-prevention trials have been negative.

[Giuliano, A.R., et al. (1998). Can cervical dysplasia and cancer be prevented with nutrients? *Nutr Rev. 1998 Jan; 56 (1 Pt 1): 9-16.* https://pubmed.ncbi.nlm.nih.gov/9481113/]

Women with high antioxidant diets were less likely to be HPV-positive initially.

Dr. Martina Barchitta and six medical colleagues at the Department of Medical and Surgical Sciences of the University of Catania in Catania Italy published an article in the May 2020 issue of the *Nutrients* journal. The article studied the benefits of dietary antioxidants and their protection against HPV infection. Diets were evaluated based on the antioxidants of zinc, selenium, manganese, vitamin A, vitamin C, vitamin E, carotenoid, and flavonoid. These doctors observed that HPV-positive women reported a decreased intake of zinc, manganese, vitamin A, and vitamin C compared to non-infected women. Women with a high antioxidant diet had lower odds of being HPV-positive. Dr. Barchitta said: "To our knowledge, this is the first study demonstrating that a diet based on the combined intake of nutrients with antioxidant properties might reduce the risk of HPV infection."

[Barchitta, M. (2020). Dietary antioxidant intake and human papillomavirus infection: evidence from a cross-sectional study in Italy. *Nutrients. 2020 May; 12 (5): 1384.* https://pubmed.ncbi.nlm.nih.gov/32408636/]

The use of beta-carotene, folic acid, and vitamin C was not shown to be of significant benefit in treating cervical dysplasia. However, one study did suggest that women with high antioxidant diets had a better chance of being HPV-negative initially, probably because their healthier immune systems could eliminate HPV infections faster.

Chapter 21
Indole-3-Carbinol Treatment for Cervical Dysplasia

S tudies with indole-3-carbinol, also called I-3-C, have had some encouraging results in treating cervical dysplasia.

Indole-3-carbinol had a benefit in the treatment of cervical dysplasia in mice.

Dr. Karen J. Auborn at the North Shore Institute for Medical Research in Manhasset New York published an article in the October 2006 issue of the *Journal of Nutrition*. Dr. Auborn found that studies with indole-3-carbinol indicate a benefit in treating cervical dysplasia and preventing cervical cancer. Dr. Auborn said: "I-3-C prevents the development of cervical cancer in this transgenic mouse. Additionally, I-3-C can reduce cervical dysplasia caused by estradiol in the normal mouse."

[Auborn, K.J. (2006). Can indole-3-carbinol-induced changes in cervical intraepithelial neoplasia be extrapolated to other food components? *J Nutr. 2006 Oct; 136 (10): 2676S-8S.* https://pubmed.ncbi.nlm.nih.gov/16988146/]

Indole-3-carbinol treatment had a 44-50% regression of cervical dysplasia at 12 weeks.

Dr. Maria C. Bell and nine medical colleagues at the Department of Obstetrics and Gynecology of Louisiana State University Medical Center in Shreveport Louisiana published an article in the August 2000 issue of the *Gynecologic Oncology* journal. They studied the use of indole-3-carbinol for cervical dysplasia. Thirty patients with biopsy-proven, moderate to severe cervical dysplasia were randomized to receive either a placebo, 200 mg per day, or 400 mg per day of indole-3-carbinol orally for 12 weeks. These doctors discovered that none of the patients in the placebo group had complete regression of cervical dysplasia. In contrast, 50% of the patients in the 200 mg per day group and 44% in the 400 mg per day group had complete regression based on their 12-week biopsy. Dr. Bell said: "There was a statistically significant regression of CIN in patients treated with I-3-C orally compared with placebo."

[Bell, M.C., et al. (2000). Placebo-controlled trial of

indole-3-carbinol in the treatment of CIN. *Gynecol Oncol. 2000 Aug; 78 (2): 123-9.* https://pubmed.ncbi.nlm.nih.gov/10926790/]

This study suggests that indole-3-carbinol is more effective than a placebo and has better success than expected from the natural history of the disease. The success was 44-50% in 3 months.

Chapter 22
AHCC Treatment for Cervical Dysplasia

A HCC is an acronym for "**A**ctive **H**exose **C**orrelated **C**ompound" which is an extract of the *Lentinula edodes* mushroom, commonly known as the Shiitake mushroom.

Dr. David Boels at the Public Health Department of Nantes University Hospital of the University of Paris in Paris France and seven medical colleagues published an article in the April 2022 issue of the journal of *Clinical Toxicology* about Shiitake mushroom dermatitis reactions reported by the Poison Control Centre in France. Dr. Boels said:

The rash appeared after Shiitake ingestion. Linear, erythematous, urticarial papules and plaques developed across the trunk, arms, and legs within a few hours and persisted for 1-40 d (median 10 d). The amount of Shiitake eaten significantly increased the duration of dermatitis. In all, 38 patients received corticosteroids, antihistamine drugs, or both without demonstrated benefit. All patients made a complete recovery. This study highlighted a dose-dependent response, suggesting a partial toxic mechanism or a Th1-type hypersensitivity mechanism. Treatment is focused on symptom management. Health professionals and the general population should be aware.

[Boels, David, et al. (2022). Shiitake dermatitis: experience of the Poison Control Centre Network in France from 2014 to 2019. *Clin Toxicol (Phila). 2022 Apr 11; 1-6.* https://pubmed.ncbi.nlm.nih.gov/35404185/]

AHCC had a 44-66% clearance of HPV at 3-7 months, but only 40.9% were still clear at 12 months.

Dr. Judith A. Smith at the Department of Obstetrics of UT Health McGovern Medical School in Houston Texas, and nine medical colleagues, published an article in the March 2019 issue of the *Frontiers in Oncology* journal. It concerned the use of AHCC in HPV infections in two small studies of women. The first study evaluated women using AHCC, 3 grams daily, from five weeks to six months. The second study evaluated women using AHCC, 1 gram daily, for eight months. Dr. Smith said:

> Four of six patients, or 66%, had confirmed HPV clearance after 3-6 months of AHCC 3 grams daily. Similarly, 4 of 9 patients, or 44%, had confirmed HPV clearance after 7 months of AHCC 1 gram daily.

[Smith, J.A., et al. (2019). From bench to bedside: evaluation of AHCC supplementation to modulate the host immunity to clear high-risk human papillomavirus infections. *Front Oncol. 2019 Mar 20; 9: 173.* https://pubmed.ncbi.nlm.nih.gov/30949451/]

Dr. Judith A. Smith at the Department of Obstetrics of UT Health McGovern Medical School in Houston Texas, and eight medical colleagues, published an article in the June 2022 issue of the *Frontiers in Oncology* journal about AHCC treatment of women with high-risk HPV. Dr. Smith found: "Fourteen of the 22 patients with AHCC supplementation were HPV-negative after 6 months."

AHCC had clearance of HPV at six months in 14 of 22 patients, or 63.6%. Only 9 of the 22 patients, or 40.9%, were still clear at 12 months.

[Smith, J.A., et al. (2022). AHCC® supplementation to support immune function to clear persistent human papillomavirus infections. *Front Oncol. 2022 Jun 22; 12: 881902.* https://pubmed.ncbi.nlm.nih.gov/35814366/]

AHCC had side effects of nausea, diarrhea, bloating, headache, fatigue, and foot cramps.

Dr. Egilius L.H. Spierings and three medical colleagues at Medvadis Research Corporation in Wellesley Hills Massachusetts published an article in the December 2007 issue of the *Journal of Nutritional Science and Vitaminology*. It was a short study on the side effects of AHCC. Twenty-six patients were in the 14-day study. Two patients dropped out of the study because of nausea and intolerance to AHCC. Six other patients experienced adverse effects of nausea, diarrhea, bloating, headache, fatigue, and foot cramps.

[Spierings, E.L.H., et al. (2007). A Phase I study of the safety of the nutritional supplement, active hexose correlated compound, AHCC, in healthy volunteers. *J Nutr Sci Vitaminol (Tokyo). 2007; Dec; 53 (6): 536-9.* https://pubmed.ncbi.nlm.nih.gov/18202543/]

These studies suggest that AHCC has similar or slightly better success than expected from the natural history of the disease. The success was 44-66% at 3-7 months but with some adverse side effects.

Chapter 23
Beta-mannan™ Treatment for
Cervical Dysplasia and Warts

Beta-mannan™ is an *Aloe vera* dietary
supplement used to treat HPV-related cervical
dysplasia and warts.

Beta-mannan™ was developed in 1996 by Dr. Joe
Glickman. He was the editor-in-chief of *Phantom
Notes*™, a series of medical books used for over twenty
years in the United States, Canada, and several other
countries to teach medical students Internal Medicine,
Surgery, Pediatrics, and Obstetrics and Gynecology.

Dr. Glickman's awareness of studies on the benefits
of *Aloe vera* prompted his examination of its effectiveness for HPV. The Beta-mannan™ website summarizes
the research that motivated this examination.

The early *Aloe vera* studies were confusing because
some showed benefits and others did not. The reason

for the mixed results eventually became clear. The studies showing effective healing were using *Aloe vera* gel that was fresh; the others were not, and the bioactive healing component in *Aloe vera* deteriorated rapidly after harvest. But when that bioactive component in the *Aloe vera* gel was fresh or preserved, it was consistently effective in healing.

The Beta-mannan™ supplement combines the best preserved, organic *Aloe vera* in a proper combination with natural Vitamin E to produce optimal healing results.

It specifically uses *Aloe vera's* polysaccharides derived from the *Aloe vera* gel which are safe, non-cytotoxic, and contain no barbaloin, the metabolite responsible for the strong laxative effect of *Aloe vera* latex. It is important to use only the *Aloe vera* gel, not the other two parts of the *Aloe vera* plant: (1) whole leaf and (2) latex. Beta-mannan™ uses the safe *Aloe vera* gel. An apple is good for you, but that doesn't mean you should eat the bark of its tree. The gel of *Aloe vera* is good for you, but that doesn't mean you should eat the rest of the plant.

[Glickman, J. (2022). *Beta-mannan™*. Beta-mannan™: Austin, Texas. Retrieved 3 July 2022 https://beta-mannan.com]

Impressed by testimonial evidence that indi-

cated a cure rate surpassing the natural history of the disease, Dr. Charles Ascher-Walsh and Dr. Jody Blanco conducted a double-blind, placebo-controlled study for cervical dysplasia patients treated with Beta-mannan™.

Dr. Charles Ascher-Walsh and Dr. Jody Blanco were two Ob-Gyn hospital staff doctors at New York Presbyterian Hospital of Columbia Medical Center in New York City:

Dr. Charles Ascher-Walsh, a nationally recognized physician, is the Director of the Division of Gynecology, Director of the Division of Urogynecology, and Director of the Division of Minimally Invasive Surgery in the Department of Obstetrics, Gynecology, and Reproductive Science at the Mount Sinai Health System. Dr. Ascher-Walsh has more than 20 years of surgical experience and has conducted extensive research with contributions to more than 100 published papers, abstracts, and textbooks relating to these conditions. His international research experience includes the completion of multiple randomized controlled trials and several projects examining minimally invasive techniques.

Dr. Ascher-Walsh has been named a Castle Connolly/*New York Magazine* Top Doctor, Most Compassionate Doctor, and a *New York Times Magazine* Super Doctor annually for the past several years. He has been a featured expert in numerous media, including *The BBC Worldwide News, New York Magazine,* and the *Huffington Post.*

[Icahn School of Medicine at Mount Sinai. (2022). *Mount Sinai.* Icahn School of Medicine at Mount Sinai: New York, New York. Retrieved 3 July 2022 https://www.mountsinai.org/profiles/charles-j-ascher-walsh]

The study designed by Dr. Ascher-Walsh and Dr. Blanco using Beta-mannan™ and a placebo lasted from January 2000 until January 2002. However, the clinic could not accumulate enough cervical dysplasia patients during the two years to complete the study. The problem: most patients chose not to risk blindly taking the placebo once they heard about the effectiveness of Beta-mannan™. They would purchase Beta-mannan™, then drop out of the study.

Still, these doctors had been impressed by the testimonials of a cure rate that significantly surpassed the natural history of the disease. Testimonials from patients of a 95% cure rate in less than three months got their attention. That is why they prepared an extensive and expensive protocol for the two-year study.

In the absence of the completed study, it is instructive to look at the kind of testimonials that motivated Dr. Ascher-Walsh and Dr. Blanco to initiate their research.

Although some of the testimonials I will cite are more recent than those that prompted the study, these are examples of the kind that got the attention of Dr. Ascher-Walsh and Dr. Blanco. Some testimonials were from traditional medical doctors. Others were from naturopathic medical practitioners who recommend Beta-mannan™ in their practices. Still, other testimonials came from Alternative Medicine websites or websites that invited stories from patients about their experiences with various remedies. Finally, some came from medical writers, most of whom had personal experience with Beta-mannan™.

Beta-mannan™ references are found on websites of traditional medical doctors.

Dr. Thomas Moraczewski at the Center for Natural and Integrative Medicine in Orlando Florida published an article in July 2012 on the website of Dr. Kirti Kalidas. Dr. Kalidas is one of few doctors both Board Certified in Internal Medicine and Licensed as a Naturopathic Physician. The article was titled *"HPV and*

Cervical Dysplasia – Alternatives to Conventional Therapy." Dr. Moraczewski, an Integrative Gynecologist Board Certified Ob-Gyn doctor, said:

> Approximately 80% of American women will become infected with HPV of the cervix by age 50. An extract from the *Aloe vera* plant called Beta-mannan™ has been reported to help eradicate cervical dysplasia by some physicians.

[Moraczewski, T. (2012). *The Center for Natural and Integrative Medicine: HPV and Cervical Dysplasia – Alternatives to Conventional Therapy.* The Center for Natural and Integrative Medicine: Orlando, Florida. Retrieved 3 July 2022 https://drkalidas.com/uncategorized/hpv-cervical-dysplasia-alternatives-to-conventional-therapy/]

Beta-mannan™ testimonials are found on websites of naturopathic doctors who recommend Beta-mannan™.

Dr. Melissa Bennett at the Olive Leaf in Atlanta Georgia is another physician who has recommended Beta-mannan™ for her patients. She is Certified as a Traditional Naturopath through the American Naturopathic Certification Board and is a Certified Natural Health Practitioner. She is Board Certified in Nutritional Wellness and has completed her accreditation as a health partner in Predictive Medicine through Emory University in Atlanta Georgia. The following is a testimonial from one of Dr. Bennett's patients:

Dear Melissa, I would like to share my testimony with you regarding my health issues. My personal experience with Beta-mannan™ was truly a wonderful success. When I came to the Olive Leaf, I was diagnosed with HPV, and I also had a 1st stage precancerous cells Pap test. Melissa Bennett, N.D., my naturopath, recommended this supplement. I contacted the company and consulted, and began to take the product as instructed. I was very nervous due to my mother dying of lung cancer and my young, 46-year-old brother dying with cancer also. I received the Beta-mannan™. I followed the instructions, which were to take the product for three months and a few other instructions, and I had a normal Pap and negative HPV test!!! Thanks so very much to Dr. Melissa Bennett for taking the time to research my very personal needs and details to find this very successful supplement. I am truly grateful and inspired. Thanks so very much!!! Nelisha.

[Bennett, M. (2022). *The Olive Leaf: Testimonials.*

The Olive Leaf: Atlanta, Georgia. Retrieved 3 July 2022 https://theoliveleaf.com/testimonials/]

Beta-mannan™ testimonials are found on websites for Alternative Medicine.

For over 20 years, *Earth Clinic,* published in Norwalk Connecticut, has been regarded as one of the top Alternative Medicine websites on the Internet. It is visited by thousands of worldwide visitors each month. On this prominent website, Leslie of Sarasota Springs in New York published an article in May 2014 titled "*Aloe* with Beta-mannan™." In this article, Leslie said:

> I was diagnosed with recurring cervical dysplasia and HPV over 10 years ago, in my early 40's. I had 3 cervical cones, where they freeze the surface cells. After the 4th positive test result, I decided to take a different action. I did a lot of online research, which led me to try a natural *Aloe*-based product known as Beta-mannan™. I took the supplement for 4 weeks along with additional Vitamin C and consciously getting more rest, more exercise, and exploring ways to de-stress. My next Pap and exam proved that I was clear, and I have never had a problem since, for over 12 years. I recommended this treatment to my sister. She was in her 30s and 2 nieces, early to mid-20s. They all

experienced the same result. Future Paps and testings were clear.

[Earth Clinic LLC. (2022). *Genital HPV Remedies: Aloe with Beta-mannan™*. Earth Clinic LLC: Norwalk, Connecticut. Retrieved 3 July 2022 https://www.earth clinic.com/cures/natural-hpv-treatment.html#bm]

Beta-mannan™ testimonials are found on websites featuring patients' experiences with various remedies.

On the *MedHelp.org* website, published by Vitals Consumer Services LLC in San Francisco California, are several testimonials about Beta-mannan™ on the page titled *"HPV, Cone Biopsy, Children, Beta-mannan™."*

Long story short, I had cervical dysplasia, moderate to high grade, had a LEEP, and all was well. I had baby number four, and 8 months later, it was back. I had moderate dysplasia and again was HPV-positive. I had decided last time around that I wanted to try a more holistic approach if there was a next time. So I ordered Beta-mannan™ and tried it for 3 months as they recommended. Went for another colposcopy, and the Beta-mannan™ had brought it down from moderate to mild... big wow! So I called the company, and they sent me ten bottles and suggested I do another 3 months. I did. I went last week for a follow-up Pap and today, I got my call. I, of course, thought it was bad news because the doctor said she would only call if there were a problem. She said that the endocervical canal and the cervical Paps were both normal! Another wow! She was really just calling to get the number to the Beta-mannan™ company for another patient. I am going to go back in 3 months for a follow-up Pap. This has truly been a blessing to me. I know that tons of women struggle with this issue, and I wish that more people knew about this supplement. Brandi.

I had HPV abnormal and found information online on Beta-mannan™ pills on my own. I had faith in Beta-mannan™ pills for three months. Took an HPV test and got the result of normal and then did an HPV test a year later, it gave me the same result normal. Rachel.

I first found out that I had an abnormal Pap smear. I went on the Internet to look up what is a remedy for HPV. Found Beta-mannan™. I tried it. I got 3 normal Pap smears in a row. I am grateful for Beta-mannan™ to prevent me from having surgeries.

[Vitals Consumer Services LLC. (2022).

MedHelp.org: HPV, Cone Biopsy, Children, Beta-mannan™. Vitals Consumer Services LLC: San Francisco, California. Retrieved 3 July 2022 https://www.medhelp.org/posts/Womens-Health/HPV-Cone-Biopsy-Children-Beta-mannan-and-now-new-problem-What-to-do/show/26690]

Beta-mannan™ testimonials are found in books by medical writers.

Andrea Segovia, in her book, *The Natural Cure for HPV*, said:

> Dr. Glickman's supplements have been sold since 1996, an all-natural *Aloe vera*-based supplement called Beta-mannan™, which has safely eliminated HPV-related illnesses in 90 days or less in the vast majority of cases for thousands of men and women who have followed the treatment recommendations with Beta-mannan™. You can take the capsules both orally and vaginally. Based on the feedback from customers since 1996, it's highly successful. Its ingredients are a nutritional food supplement, and it contains a very specific combination of extracts and concentrates of the healing compounds found in *Aloe vera*. It is completely natural and organic.

[Segovia, Andrea. (2022). *The Natural Cure for HPV*.

pp. 15-24. Retrieved 3 July 2022 https://bit.ly/natural cureforhpv]

Zayna de Gaia, in her book, *Thank You for HPV*, made a reference to Beta-mannan™ as the essential ingredient in her eradication of HPV. Zayna said:

This is the magic ingredient to this healing formula. Everything else in this chapter can and will keep anyone super healthy and feeling great, but the Beta-mannan™ is specific to the condition of HPV. Dr. Joe Glickman created an all-natural *Aloe vera*-based supplement called Beta-mannan™, which has safely eliminated HPV-related illnesses in 90 days or less in the vast majority of cases for thousands of men and women who have followed the treatment recommendations with Beta-mannan™, including myself. Its ingredients are a nutritional food supplement, and it contains a very specific combination of extracts and concentrates of the healing compounds found in *Aloe vera*. It is completely natural and organic. You can take the capsules both orally and vaginally. This supplement played a vital part in me being HPV-free. It's the key element for healing HPV.

[de Gaia, Zayna. (2013). *Thank You for HPV, pp. 64-65.*]

Kimberly Dedes provides a detailed description of how to use Beta-mannan™ in her article on the *eHow* website, published by the Leaf Group Ltd in Santa Monica California.

> Take one pill four times daily. Use a Beta-mannan™ capsule as a suppository twice daily, morning and evening, unless menstruating, to coat the cervix and vaginal walls. Do this in addition to taking the substance orally if you intend to use the product to aid with an existing cervical dysplasia or a vaginal HPV infection. Continue taking the supplement for 90 days.

[Leaf Group Ltd. (2022). *eHow: How to take Beta-mannan™*. Leaf Group Ltd: Santa Monica California. Retrieved 3 July 2022 https://www.ehow.co.uk/how_8574055_beta-mannan.html]

Beta-mannan™ is a food supplement, not a drug.

The supplement industry often points out that obtaining FDA approval for a drug is an expensive and lengthy process. It averages twelve years, an application of 100,000 pages and a cost of one billion dollars. Only after this process and approval does the FDA allow a manufacturer to claim the drug targets a specific illness.

[Williams, S. (2018). *The Motley Fool: The cost of developing an FDA-approved drug is truly staggering, studies show.* The Motley Fool: Alexandria, Virginia. Retrieved 3 July 2022 https://www.fool.com/investing/general/2016/04/30/the-cost-of-developing-an-fda-approved-drug-is-tru.aspx]

Beta-mannan™ has not been through this extensive process. So when testimonials of Beta-mannan™ effectiveness were posted on the Beta-mannan™ website, the FDA warned that such claims are not allowed. The testimonials were removed from the website, and since 2008 none have been posted there.

The following summarizes what the testimonials about Beta-mannan™ say about its effectiveness, treatment regimen, and daily use.

Beta-mannan™ is effective.

It can be considered an effective alternative therapy for HPV, more effective than expected from the natural history of cervical dysplasia or warts.

A great many testimonials support the effectiveness of Beta-mannan™ against the HPV-related diseases of cervical dysplasia and warts. Beta-mannan™ has produced consistent results without side effects in both men and women. Treatment with this low-cost natural therapy should be considered for cervical dysplasia and warts.

Women who tested positive for HPV before Beta-mannan™ therapy have tested negative for HPV after 90 days of treatment in over 95% of cases.

The natural history of HPV would predict a 70% cure rate in 2 years, whereas Beta-mannan™ has a 95% cure rate in 3 months.

Surgical treatments do not seem logical for an infection such as cervical dysplasia unless cancer is present. Beta-mannan™ treatment is superior to surgical procedures. When long-term results are compared, the surgical procedures for HPV are uncomfortable, expensive, and less effective. Beta-mannan™, in contrast, is painless, inexpensive, and more effective.

The treatment regimen for Beta-mannan™ is straightforward.

For cervical dysplasia: Beta-mannan™ should be taken orally, four capsules daily, and used vaginally as a suppository, one capsule twice daily, morning and evening, except during menses, for 90 days. This requires three bottles of Beta-mannan™ per month.

For warts: Beta-mannan™ should be taken orally, four capsules daily, and applied topically to a wart, one capsule twice daily, for 90 days. Gently file at least one wart daily with a fingernail file. Apply Beta-mannan™

to the filed wart. No filing should be done on facial warts. Only one wart needs to be treated with filing since all the other warts will disappear once immunity develops. This requires three bottles of Beta-mannan™ per month.

For cervical dysplasia and warts: Beta-mannan™ should be taken orally, four capsules daily, and used vaginally as a suppository, one capsule twice daily, morning and evening, except during menses, and applied topically to a wart, one capsule twice daily, for 90 days. Gently file at least one wart daily with a finger-nail file. Apply Beta-mannan™ to the filed wart. No filing should be done on facial warts. Only one wart needs to be treated with filing since all the other warts will disappear once immunity develops. This requires four bottles of Beta-mannan™ per month.

Many recommend Beta-mannan™ for daily immune support.

For good health maintenance: Beta-mannan™ should be taken orally, two capsules daily, and used vaginally as a suppository, one capsule weekly, except during menses. This requires one bottle of Beta-mannan™ per month.

Maintenance use of Beta-mannan™ helps maintain a strong immune system. When exposed to other HPV types, you are more likely to develop immunity faster to the new types before they cause symptoms and before they are detected if you are already taking Beta-mannan™. HPV-negative tests do not rule out an HPV infection because (1) less than 10% of the known 228 HPV types are usually tested, and (2) the tests can yield false-negative results even for the few types tested.

After treatment, follow-up by a qualified health care professional is recommended to confirm the effectiveness of the therapy.

Chapter 24
Aloe Vera Benefits for the Immune System and Various Conditions

Considering the success of Beta-mannan™ for HPV treatment, it may be interesting to review other research about *Aloe vera,* a key ingredient of Beta-mannan™.

Many of you have probably heard about the healing benefits of *Aloe vera* but wondered how scientifically proven they are. I want to digress in this chapter to provide facts about the general uses of *Aloe vera* throughout history and in modern science.

This will not only satisfy the curiosity of those who want to know more about *Aloe vera* but also help explain why *Aloe vera* apparently is beneficial in addressing HPV.

Aloe vera is also known by its botanical name of *Aloe barbadensis miller.*

Aloe vera **has been used for medicinal purposes for at least 4,000 years. It was highly valued in ancient Greece and Egypt.**

The Greeks regarded *Aloe vera* as the panacea for all medical conditions. The Egyptians believed it was the plant necessary for immortality.

[Surjushe, A., et al. (2008). *Aloe vera:* a short review. *Indian J Dermatol. 2008; 53 (4): 163–166.* https://www.ncbi.nlm.nih.gov/pmc/articles/PMC2763764/]

Interesting historical fact: Alexander the Great and Christopher Columbus used *Aloe vera* for wound healing.

Dr. Mariko Moriyama at the Pharmaceutical Research and Technology Institute of Kindai University in Osaka Japan, and nine medical colleagues, published an article in the October 2016 issue of the *Public Library of Science* journal about the beneficial effects of *Aloe vera*. According to these doctors, Cleopatra used *Aloe vera* for her skin, and Alexander the Great and Christopher Columbus used *Aloe vera* to treat wounds. Dr. Moriyama said:

The genus *Aloe* comprises about 600 species. However, only a few species of *Aloe*, including *Aloe vera* and *Cape Aloe*, have been reported to contain many bioactive ingredients. *Aloe vera* is the most commercialized of all *Aloe* species.

[Moriyama, M., et al. (2016). Beneficial effects of the genus *Aloe* on wound healing, cell proliferation, and differentiation of epidermal keratinocytes. *PLoS One. 2016; 11 (10): e0164799.* https://www.ncbi.nlm.nih.gov/pmc/articles/PMC5063354/]

We will cover these 23 facts about *Aloe vera*.

(1) *Aloe vera* has been used worldwide as a medicinal plant to treat various diseases.

(2) *Aloe vera* activates the immune system against influenza viral infections.

(3) *Aloe vera* restores an immune system damaged by stress.

(4) *Aloe vera* stimulates the immune system's natural killer cell activity against cancer cells.

(5) *Aloe vera* suppresses colon cancer by inhibiting chronic inflammation.

(6) *Aloe vera* cured cancer on the cornea of the eye.

(7) *Aloe vera* has antimicrobial effects against various bacteria, including *Staphylococcus aureus*. These antimicrobial effects were as strong as those of ofloxacin and ciprofloxacin, potent antibiotics.

(8) *Aloe vera* has antimicrobial effects against

antibiotic-resistant strains of *Helicobacter pylori*, the bacteria that can cause stomach ulcers.

(9) *Aloe vera* reduces cigarette smoke-induced lung damage.

(10) *Aloe vera* has anti-inflammatory properties that help gastroesophageal reflux disease.

(11) *Aloe vera* has anti-inflammatory properties that help irritable bowel syndrome.

(12) *Aloe vera* has anti-inflammatory properties that help inflammatory bowel disease.

(13) *Aloe vera* has anti-inflammatory properties that help active ulcerative colitis in 30-47% of patients.

(14) *Aloe vera* has anti-inflammatory properties that help rheumatoid arthritis and the chronic pain of osteoarthritis.

(15) *Aloe vera* has anti-inflammatory properties that help multiple sclerosis.

(16) *Aloe vera* has anti-inflammatory properties that help food allergies and allergic rhinitis.

(17) *Aloe vera* has anti-inflammatory properties that help hypothyroidism in 100% of patients.

(18) *Aloe vera* is equal to chlorhexidine mouthwash for treating periodontal disease but without the side effects.

(19) *Aloe vera's* polysaccharides derived from the *Aloe vera* gel are safe, non-cytotoxic, and contain no

barbaloin, the metabolite responsible for the strong laxative effect of *Aloe vera* latex. It is important to use only the *Aloe vera* gel, not the other two parts of the *Aloe* plant: (1) whole leaf and (2) latex. Beta-mannan™ uses the safe *Aloe vera* gel. An apple is good for you, but that doesn't mean you should eat the bark of its tree. The gel of *Aloe vera* is good for you, but that doesn't mean you should eat the rest of the plant.

(20) *Aloe vera* life-long ingestion in rats prevents age-related diseases and does not cause harmful side effects.

(21) *Aloe vera* significantly improves skin appearance by increasing skin elasticity, hydration, and collagen score in healthy women. This was proven by ultrasound echogenicity. These results suggest that continued *Aloe vera* ingestion contributes to maintaining healthy skin.

(22) *Aloe vera* decreases fasting blood glucose and improves lipid profiles in pre-diabetics.

(23) *Aloe vera* decreases fasting blood glucose and improves lipid profiles in type II diabetics and heart disease patients. It reverses angina pectoris symptoms and associated ECG changes.

Let's take a closer look now at these 23 important facts and the studies that support them.

(1) *Aloe vera* has been used worldwide as a medi-

cinal plant to treat various diseases.

Dr. Ramesh Kumar at the Department of Biochemistry of the University of Allahabad in Uttar Pradesh India, and four medical colleagues, published an article in the July 2019 issue of the *Phytomedicine* journal. Dr. Kumar noted:

> *Aloe vera* is commonly used in the primary health care of human beings since time immemorial. It is an herb widely used in various traditional systems of medicine worldwide. Systematic and scientific investigation of *Aloe vera* as a medicinal plant has drawn considerable attention, and many laboratories are involved in the isolation, characterization, and evaluation of phyto-constituents for their nutraceutical and pharmaceutical applications. Various biological and pharmacological activities of *Aloe vera*, such as antioxidant, anti-inflammatory, immunomodulatory, antimicrobial, antiviral, anti-diabetic, hepatoprotective, anticancer, skin-protective, and wound-healing responses, have been attributed to the presence of many active compounds, including anthraquinones, anthrones, chromones, flavonoids, amino acids, lipids, carbohydrates, vitamins, and minerals. Based on

various preclinical studies, *Aloe vera* constituents have enormous potential to prevent and treat various diseases.

[Kumar, R., et al. (2019). Therapeutic potential of *Aloe vera* - A miracle gift of nature. *Phytomedicine. 2019 Jul; 60: 152996.* https://pubmed.ncbi.nlm.nih.gov/31272819/]

(2) ***Aloe vera* activates the immune system against influenza viral infections.**

Dr. Zhenhong Sun at the School of Basic Medical Sciences of Taishan Medical University in Tai'an China, and seven medical colleagues, published an article in the September 2018 issue of the *Frontiers of Microbiology* journal. Dr. Sun noted that their previous studies have shown that certain extracts of *Aloe vera* can increase the activity of the immune system, which is an essential mechanism against viral infections, including influenza A. Dr. Sun said:

> *Aloe vera* directly interacted with influenza virus particles. *Aloe vera* considerably ameliorated the clinical symptoms and the lung damage of the infected mice, and significantly reduced the virus loads and mortality.

[Sun, Z., et al. (2018). *Aloe* polysaccharides inhibit influenza A virus infection - a promising natural anti-flu drug. *Front Microbiol. 2018; 9: 2338.* https://www.ncbi.nlm.nih.gov/pmc/articles/PMC6170609/]

(3) ***Aloe vera*** **restores an immune system damaged by stress.**

Dr. Youngjoo Lee at the College of Pharmacy of Sahmyook University in Seoul South Korea, and eleven medical colleagues, published an article in the October 2016 issue of the *International Journal of Molecular Sciences. Aloe vera* was found to restore an immune system damaged by stress in mice. They pointed out that chronic stress suppresses the immune system of humans and makes them more vulnerable to disease. Dr. Lee found that *Aloe vera* restored the activities of lymphocytes and antibody production, thereby significantly reducing the damage caused by stress-induced immunosuppression. Dr. Lee said:

> Chronic stress, generally experienced in our daily lives, is known to augment disease vulnerability by suppressing the host immune system. Oral administration of *Aloe* ameliorated chronic stress-induced immunosuppression.

[Lee, Y., et al. (2016). Modified *Aloe* polysaccharide restores chronic stress-induced immunosuppression in mice. *Int J Mol Sci. 2016 Oct; 17 (10): 1660.* https://www.ncbi.nlm.nih.gov/pmc/articles/PMC5085693/]

(4) *Aloe vera* **stimulates the immune system's natural killer cell activity against cancer cells.**

Dr. Ioannis Toliopoulos at the Laboratory of Physiology of the Medical School of the University of Ioannina in Ioannina Greece, and four medical colleagues, published an article in the June 2012 issue of the *Journal of Herbal Medicine*. Dr. Toliopoulos found natural killer cell stimulation against cancer cells with *Aloe vera* and vitamin C and said: "These results indicate that vitamin C and *Aloe vera* juice can modulate natural killer cells cytotoxicity and has the potential to enhance the immune system."

[Toliopoulos, I., et al. (2012). NK cell stimulation by administration of vitamin C and *Aloe vera* juice in vitro and in vivo: A pilot study. *J Herbal Medicine. 2012 June; 2 (2): 29-33.* https://www.sciencedirect.com/science/article/abs/pii/S2210803312000371]

(5) *Aloe vera* **suppresses colon cancer by inhibiting chronic inflammation.**

Dr. Sun-A Im at the College of Pharmacy of Chungbuk National University in Cheongju South

Korea, and seven medical colleagues, published an article in the November 2016 issue of the *International Immunopharmacology* journal. *Aloe vera* was found to suppress colon cancer in mice. Dr. Im discovered: "These findings show that *Aloe vera* gel suppresses colitis-related colon carcinogenesis by inhibiting both chronic inflammation and cell cycle progression in the colon."

[Im, S., et al. (2016). Prevention of azoxymethane/dextran sodium sulfate-induced mouse colon carcinogenesis by processed *Aloe vera* gel. *Int Immunopharmacol. 2016 Nov; 40: 428-435.* https://pubmed.ncbi.nlm.nih.gov/27697726/]

(6) *Aloe vera* **cured cancer on the cornea of the eye.**

Dr. Mausam R. Damani at the Department of Ophthalmology of the University of Pennsylvania in Philadelphia Pennsylvania, and three medical colleagues, published an article in the January 2015 issue of the *Cornea* journal. They discussed a case of cancer on the surface of the eye's cornea of a 64-year-old woman. She was treated successfully with *Aloe vera* drops three times daily. Dr. Damani said:

The patient refused biopsy of her lesion and traditional treatments and, instead, initiated using *Aloe vera* eye drops 3 times daily. At follow-up visits, the lesion was noted to regress until it finally resolved 3 months after commencing treatment. No additional topical medications were used, and she has remained tumor-free for 6 years.

[Damani, M.R., et al. (2015). Treatment of ocular surface squamous neoplasia with topical *Aloe vera* drops. *Cornea. 2015 Jan; 34 (1): 87-9.* https://pubmed. ncbi.nlm.nih.gov/25393094/]

(7) *Aloe vera* **has antimicrobial effects against various bacteria, including** *Staphylococcus aureus.* **These antimicrobial effects were as strong as those of ofloxacin and ciprofloxacin, potent antibiotics.**

Dr. Supreet Jain at the Department of Oral Medicine and Radiology of New Horizon Dental College in Chhattisgarh India, and seven medical colleagues, published an article in the November 2016 issue of the *Journal of Clinical and Diagnostic Research*. Dr. Jain found antibacterial effects of *Aloe vera* against oral pathogens and said:

Natural herbal remedies have shown promising antimicrobial properties and fewer side effects compared to synthetic antimicrobial therapy. *Aloe vera* is a medicinal plant used for management of various infections since ancient times as it has anti-inflamma-tory, antimicrobial, and immune-boosting properties.

In this study, Dr. Jain measured the antimicrobial effects of *Aloe vera* against a variety of oral bacteria, including *Staphylococcus aureus*. With high concentrations of *Aloe vera*, he obtained a result against the bacteria equally as impressive as with the potent antibiotics of ofloxacin and ciprofloxacin.

[Jain, S., et al. (2016). Antibacterial effect of *Aloe vera* gel against oral pathogens: An in-vitro study. *J Clin Diagn Res. 2016 Nov; 10 (11): ZC41-ZC44*. https://pubmed.ncbi.nlm.nih.gov/28050502/]

(8) *Aloe vera* has antimicrobial effects against antibiotic-resistant strains of *Helicobacter pylori*, the bacteria that can cause stomach ulcers.

Dr. L. Cellini and five medical colleagues at the Department of Pharmacy of the University G. d'Annunzio Chieti-Pescara in Chieti Italy published an article in the July 2014 issue of the *Letters of Applied Microbiology* journal. *Aloe vera* gel had antibacterial effects against *H. pylori* strains that are resistant to antibiotics. Dr. Cellini said:

The study demonstrates that the *Aloe vera* inner gel expresses antibacterial properties against susceptible and resistant *Helicobacter pylori* strains. These findings may impact on the antimicrobial resistance phenomenon of *H. pylori*, proposing the *Aloe vera* inner gel as a novel effective natural agent for combination with antibiotics for the treatment of *H. pylori* gastric infection.

[Cellini, L., et al. (2014). In vitro activity of *Aloe vera* inner gel against *Helicobacter pylori* strains. *Lett Appl Microbiol. 2014 Jul; 59 (1): 43-8.* https://pubmed.ncbi. nlm.nih.gov/24597562/]

(9) *Aloe vera* **reduces cigarette smoke-induced lung damage.**

Dr. Ashwani Koul and three medical colleagues at the Department of Biophysics of Panjab University in Chandigarh India published an article in the September 2015 issue of the journal of *Environmental Toxicology. Aloe vera* was found to reduce cigarette smoke-induced lung damage in mice. Cigarette smoke inhalation for four weeks caused significant lung damage in the control group that was not treated with *Aloe vera*. However, lung damage was significantly less in the group treated with *Aloe vera*. Dr. Koul said:

These observations suggest that *Aloe vera* has the potential to modulate cigarette smoke-induced changes in the pulmonary tissue, which could have implications in the management of cigarette smoke-associated pulmonary diseases.

[Koul, A., et al. (2015). *Aloe vera* affects changes induced in pulmonary tissue of mice caused by cigarette smoke inhalation. *Environ Toxicol. 2015 Sep; 30 (9): 999-1013.* https://pubmed.ncbi.nlm.nih.gov/24615921/]

(10) *Aloe vera* has anti-inflammatory properties that help gastroesophageal reflux disease.

Dr. Yunes Panahi at the Chemical Injuries Research Center of Baqiyatallah University of Medical Sciences in Tehran Iran, and four medical colleagues, published an article in the December 2015 issue of the *Journal of Traditional Chinese Medicine. Aloe vera* was found to reduce symptoms of gastroesophageal reflux disease, also called GERD. The study consisted of 79 patients. Dr. Panahi said:

> The frequencies of eight main symptoms of GERD, namely heartburn, food regurgitation, flatulence, belching, dysphagia, nausea, vomiting, and acid regurgitation, were assessed at weeks 2 and 4 of the trial. *Aloe vera* was safe and well-tolerated and reduced the frequencies of all the assessed GERD

symptoms, with no adverse events requiring withdrawal. *Aloe vera* may provide a safe and effective treatment for reducing the symptoms of GERD.

[Panahi, Y., et al. (2015). Efficacy and safety of *Aloe vera* syrup for the treatment of gastroesophageal reflux disease: a pilot randomized positive-controlled trial. *J Tradit Chin Med. 2015 Dec; 35 (6): 632-6.* https://pubmed.ncbi.nlm.nih.gov/26742306/]

(11) *Aloe vera* has anti-inflammatory properties that help irritable bowel syndrome.

Dr. Stine Storsrud at the Department of Internal Medicine of the University of Gothenburg in Gothenburg Sweden, and two medical colleagues, published an article in the September 2015 issue of the *Journal of Gastrointestinal and Liver Diseases. Aloe vera* was found to improve irritable bowel syndrome. Dr. Storsrud said: "The overall severity of the gastrointestinal symptoms was reduced in the *Aloe vera* group but not the placebo group."

[Storsrud, S., et al. (2015). A pilot study of the effect of *Aloe barbadensis miller* extract (AVH200®) in patients with irritable bowel syndrome: A randomized, double-blind, placebo-controlled study. *J Gastrointestin Liver Dis. 2015 Sep; 24 (3): 275-80.* https://pubmed.ncbi.nlm.nih.gov/26405698/]

(12) *Aloe vera* has anti-inflammatory properties that help inflammatory bowel disease.

Dr. L. Langmead at the Centre for Adult and Paediatric Gastroenterology of Barts and Queen Mary School of Medicine and Dentistry in London England, and two medical colleagues, published an article in the March 2004 issue of the *Alimentary Pharmacology and Therapeutics* journal. *Aloe vera* was found to have anti-inflammatory effects on the mucosa of the colon. Dr. Langmead noted that *Aloe vera* is widely used for inflammatory bowel disease. Dr. Langmead said: "The anti-inflammatory actions of *Aloe vera* gel in vitro provide support for the proposal that it may have a therapeutic effect in inflammatory bowel disease."

[Langmead, L., et al. (2004). Anti-inflammatory effects of *Aloe vera* gel in human colorectal mucosa in vitro. *Aliment Pharmacol Ther. 2004 Mar 1; 19 (5): 521-7.* https://pubmed.ncbi.nlm.nih.gov/14987320/]

(13) *Aloe vera* has anti-inflammatory properties that help active ulcerative colitis in 30-47% of patients.

Dr. L. Langmead at the Centre for Adult and Paediatric Gastroenterology of Barts and Queen Mary School of Medicine and Dentistry in London England, and two medical colleagues, published an article in the April 2005 issue of the *Alimentary Pharmacology and Thera-*

peutics journal. *Aloe vera* was shown to benefit active ulcerative colitis. These doctors found that clinical improvement occurred in 30-47% receiving the *Aloe vera* compared to 7-14% receiving the placebo. Dr. Langmead concluded: "Oral *Aloe vera* taken for 4 weeks produced a clinical response more often than placebo; it also reduced the histological disease activity and appeared safe."

[Langmead, L., et al. (2004). Randomized, double-blind, placebo-controlled trial of oral *Aloe vera* gel for active ulcerative colitis. *Aliment Pharmacol Ther. 2004 Apr 1; 19 (7): 739-47.* https://pubmed.ncbi.nlm.nih.gov/15043514/]

(14) *Aloe vera* has anti-inflammatory properties that help rheumatoid arthritis and the chronic pain of osteoarthritis.

Dr. Motoko Hashiguchi at the Department of Medicine of Juntendo University Graduate School of Medicine in Tokyo Japan, and three medical colleagues, published an article in the June 2017 issue of the *Molecular Medicine Reports* journal. *Aloe vera* was described as a potential therapy for rheumatoid arthritis. Dr. Hashiguchi found that *Aloe vera*:

May be a potential therapeutic agent for the treatment of rheumatoid arthritis, and may be complementary to methotrexate, based on its anti-proliferative effect on synovial cells.

[Hashiguchi, M., et al. (2017). Effect of *Aloe*-emodin on the proliferation and apoptosis of human synovial MH7A cells; a comparison with methotrexate. *Mol Med Rep. 2017 Jun; 15 (6): 4398-4404.* https://pubmed.ncbi. nlm.nih.gov/28487948/]

Dr. David Cowan at the Institute for Strategic Leadership and Service Improvement of the Faculty of Health of London South Bank University in London England published an article in the June 2010 issue of the *British Journal of Community Nursing*. Dr. Cowan said: "Oral *Aloe vera* could be used in the treatment of chronic non-cancer pain, particularly that caused by osteoarthritis."

[Cowan, D. (2010). Oral *Aloe vera* as a treatment for osteoarthritis: a summary. *Br J Community Nurs. 2010 Jun; 15 (6): 280-2.* https://pubmed.ncbi.nlm.nih.gov/ 20679979/]

(15) *Aloe vera* has anti-inflammatory properties that help multiple sclerosis.

Dr. A. Mirshafiey and six medical colleagues at the Department of Immunology of Tehran University of Medical Sciences in Tehran Iran published an article in the September 2010 issue of the journal of

Immunopharmacology and Immunotoxicology. Aloe vera was shown to reduce the severity of multiple sclerosis. Dr. Mirshafiey found the following:

> The results indicated that treatment with *Aloe vera* caused a significant reduction in the severity of the disease in our experimental model of multiple sclerosis. These data indicate that *Aloe vera* therapy can attenuate the disease progression in an experimental model of multiple sclerosis.

[Mirshafiey, A., et al. (2010). Therapeutic approach by *Aloe vera* in experimental model of multiple sclerosis. *Immunopharmacology and Immunotoxicology*. 2010 Sep; 32 (3): 410-5. https://pubmed.ncbi.nlm.nih.gov/20233107/]

(16) *Aloe vera* has anti-inflammatory properties that help food allergies and allergic rhinitis.

Dr. Dajeong Lee at the Department of Immunology of the College of Medicine of Konkuk University in Chungju South Korea, and thirteen medical colleagues, published an article in the February 2018 issue of the *Biomedicine and Pharmacotherapy* journal about *Aloe vera* treatment for food allergies. Dr. Lee said:

Food allergy is a hypersensitive immune reaction to food proteins and the number of patients with food allergy has recently increased. *Aloe vera* is used for wellness and medicinal purposes. In particular, *Aloe vera* has been reported to enhance immunity. In this study, we investigated the effects of processed *Aloe vera* gel on ovalbumin-induced food allergy in mice. *Aloe vera* suppressed the decrease of body temperature, diarrhea, and allergic symptoms in food allergy mice.

[Lee, D., et al. (2018). Polysaccharide isolated from *Aloe vera* gel suppresses ovalbumin-induced food allergy through inhibition of Th2 immunity in mice. *Biomed Pharmacother. 2018 May; 101: 201-210.* https://pubmed.ncbi.nlm.nih.gov/29494957/]

Dr. Hongwei Yu and two medical colleagues at the Department of Otolaryngology of Jilin University in Changchun China published an article in the May 2002 issue of the *Journal of Clinical Otorhinolaryngology* about *Aloe vera* and allergic rhinitis. Dr. Yu said:

Ovalbumin-sensitized white rat used as animal models of allergic rhinitis were treated intra-nasally with *Aloe vera*. Inflammatory reactions in the experimental group nasal mucosa were remarkably relieved.

The results suggests that local *Aloe vera* treatment was a selective and non-traumatic method to treat the allergic rhinitis.

[Yu, H., et al. (2002). Molecular biological study of *Aloe vera* in the treatment of experimental allergic rhinitis in the rat. *Lin Chuang Er Bi Yan Hou Ke Za Zhi. 2002 May; 16 (5): 229-31.* https://pubmed.ncbi.nlm.nih.gov/12592663/]

(17) *Aloe vera* has anti-inflammatory properties that help hypothyroidism in 100% of patients.

Dr. Daniela Metro at the Department of Biomedical and Dental Sciences of the University of Messina in Messina Italy, and three medical colleagues, published an article in the March 2018 issue of the *Journal of Clinical and Translational Endocrinology*. *Aloe vera* was shown to restore thyroid function in patients with subclinical hypothyroidism. Of the thirty women enrolled in the study with subclinical hypothyroidism who took *Aloe vera,* 100% had normal values in nine months. In contrast, none of the fifteen women in the control group who took the placebo had any improvement.

[Metro, D., et al. (2018). Marked improvement of thyroid function and autoimmunity by *Aloe barbadensis miller* juice was shown in patients with subclinical hypothyroidism. *J Clin Transl Endocrinol. 2018 Mar; 11: 18–25.* https://www.ncbi.nlm.nih.gov/pmc/articles/ PMC5842288/]

(18) *Aloe vera* **is equal to chlorhexidine mouthwash for treating periodontal disease but without the side effects.**

Dr. Bushra Karim at the Department of Public Health Dentistry of Teerthankar Mahaveer Dental College in Uttar Pradesh India, and six medical colleagues, published an article in the March 2014 issue of the *Oral Health and Dental Management* journal. *Aloe vera* was shown to benefit periodontal disease. Dr. Karim said:

> Our result showed that *Aloe vera* mouth rinse is equally effective in reducing periodontal indices as chlorhexidine. The results demonstrated a significant reduction of gingival bleeding and plaque indices in both groups over a period of 15 and 30 days as compared to the placebo group. There was a significant reduction in plaque and gingivitis in *Aloe vera* and chlorhexidine groups, and no statistically significant difference was observed among them. *Aloe vera* mouthwash showed no side effects, as seen with chlorhexidine. The results of the present study indicate that *Aloe vera* may prove to be an effective mouth-

wash owing to its ability in reducing periodontal indices.

[Karim, B., et al. (2014). Effect of *Aloe vera* mouthwash on periodontal health: triple blind randomized control trial. *Oral Health Dent Manag. 2014 Mar; 13 (1): 14-9.* https://pubmed.ncbi.nlm.nih.gov/24603910/]

(19) ***Aloe vera's* polysaccharides derived from the *Aloe vera* gel are safe, non-cytotoxic, and contain no barbaloin, the metabolite responsible for the strong laxative effect of *Aloe vera* latex. It is important to use only the *Aloe vera* gel, not the other two parts of the *Aloe* plant: (1) whole leaf and (2) latex. Beta-mannan™ uses the safe *Aloe vera* gel. An apple is good for you, but that doesn't mean you should eat the bark of its tree. The gel of *Aloe vera* is good for you, but that doesn't mean you should eat the rest of the plant.**

Dr. Xiaoqing Guo and Dr. Nan Mei at the Division of Genetic and Molecular Research in Jefferson Arkansas published an article in the April 2016 issue of the *Journal of Environmental Science and Health* about the three parts of the *Aloe vera* plant in respect to their safety and toxicity. Dr. Guo said:

Aloe plant contains multiple constituents with potential beneficial and toxicological activities. Three distinct preparations are derived from *Aloe vera*: (1) the whole leaf extract, (2) *Aloe vera* gel, and (3) *Aloe vera* latex. They have been used as topical and oral therapeutic remedies. The gel is primarily used topically for wounds and skin problems, as well as taken orally for the treatment of gastrointestinal ulcers and diabetes. The latex is regulated as a drug by the FDA to relieve constipation, and the whole leaf extract may possess antibacterial/viral and anticancer activities. *Aloe vera* appears to be safe when used as a flavoring in foods; and the polysaccharide material derived from the inner gel is non-cytotoxic as evaluated by the Cosmetic Ingredient Review Expert Panel.

[Guo, X., et al. (2019). Aloe vera: A review of toxicity and adverse clinical effects. *J Environ Sci Health Rev. 2016 Apr 2; 34 (2): 77–96.* https://www.ncbi.nlm.nih.gov/pmc/articles/PMC6349368/]

Dr. Mariko Moriyama at the Pharmaceutical Research and Technology Institute of Kindai University in Osaka Japan, and nine medical colleagues, published an article in the October 2016 issue of the *Public Library of Science* journal about the beneficial effects of *Aloe vera*. According to these doctors:

Aloe vera gel contains no barbaloin, a metabolite responsible for the strong laxative effect of *Aloe*. Therefore, *Aloe vera* gel has been used as an ingredient in food products and for the production of gel-containing health drinks and yogurt.

[Moriyama, M., et al. (2016). Beneficial effects of the genus *Aloe* on wound healing, cell proliferation, and differentiation of epidermal keratinocytes. *PLoS One. 2016; 11 (10): e0164799.* https://www.ncbi.nlm.nih.gov/pmc/articles/PMC5063354/]

(20) *Aloe vera* life-long ingestion in rats prevents age-related diseases and does not cause harmful side effects.

Dr. Yuji Ikeno and four medical colleagues at the Department of Physiology of the University of Texas Health Science Center in San Antonio Texas published an article in the December 2002 issue of the *Physiotherapy Research* journal regarding the effect of long-term *Aloe vera* ingestion on age-related diseases in rats. Dr. Ikeno found that the groups given *Aloe vera* exhibited significantly less occurrence of multiple causes of death, a slightly lower incidence of fatal chronic nephropathy, and slightly lower incidences of thrombosis in the cardiac atrium. Dr. Ikeno said:

This study demonstrates that life-long *Aloe vera* ingestion produced neither harmful effects nor deleterious changes. In addition, *Aloe vera* ingestion appeared to be associated with some beneficial effects on age-related diseases. Therefore, these findings suggest that life-long *Aloe vera* ingestion does not cause any obvious harmful and deleterious side effects and could also be beneficial for the prevention of age-related pathology.

[Ikeno, Y., et al. (2002). The influence of long-term *Aloe vera* ingestion on age-related disease in male Fischer 344 rats. *Phytother Res. 2002 Dec; 16 (8): 712-8.* https://pubmed.ncbi.nlm.nih.gov/12458471/]

(21) ***Aloe vera*** **significantly improves skin appearance by increasing skin elasticity, hydration, and collagen score in healthy women. This was proven by ultrasound echogenicity. These results suggest that continued *Aloe vera* ingestion contributes to maintaining healthy skin.**

Dr. Miyuki Tanaka and seven medical colleagues at the Functional Food Ingredients Department of the Food Ingredients and Technology Institute in Zama City Japan published an article in the 2016 issue of the journal of *Skin Pharmacology and Physiology*. *Aloe vera* was proven to help maintain healthy skin. These doctors performed a 12-week study to evaluate the effects of oral *Aloe* supplementation on skin elasticity, hydration, and collagen score in 64 healthy women ages 30-59. The gross elasticity, net elasticity, and biological elasticity scores of the *Aloe* group significantly increased with time. Dr. Tanaka said:

In addition, skin fatigue area F3, which is known to decrease with age and fatigue, also increased with *Aloe* sterol intake. Ultrasound echogenicity revealed that the collagen content in the dermis increased with *Aloe* sterol intake. The results suggest that continued *Aloe* sterol ingestion contributes to maintaining healthy skin.

[Tanaka, M., et al. (2016). Effects of *Aloe* sterol supplementation on skin elasticity, hydration, and collagen score: A 12-week double-blind, randomized, controlled trial. *Skin Pharmacol Physiol. 2016; 29 (6): 309-317.* https://pubmed.ncbi.nlm.nih.gov/28088806/]

(22) *Aloe vera* decreases fasting blood glucose and improves lipid profiles in pre-diabetics.

Dr. Samaneh Alinejad-Mofrad at the Faculty of Nursing and Midwifery of Birjand University of Medical Sciences in Birjand Iran, and three medical colleagues, published an article in the April 2015 issue of the

Journal of Diabetes and Metabolic Disorders. Aloe vera decreased fasting blood glucose and triglycerides in pre-diabetics after 4-8 weeks. HbA1C, total cholesterol, LDL-C, and HDL-C levels were significantly improved after eight weeks of using *Aloe vera.*

[Alinejad-Mofrad, S., et al. (2015). Improvement of glucose and lipid profile status with *Aloe vera* in pre-diabetic subjects: a randomized controlled trial. *J Diabetes Metab Disord. 2015 Apr 9; 14: 22.* https:// pubmed.ncbi.nlm.nih.gov/25883909/]

Dr. Yiyi Zhang at the Department of Endocrinology and Metabolism of Sichuan University in Chengdu China, and four medical colleagues, published an article in the July 2016 issue of the *Nutrients* journal. Their studies consisted of 415 patients. *Aloe vera* decreased fasting blood glucose and improved lipid profiles in pre-diabetic patients and early non-treated diabetic patients. Fasting blood glucose levels were significantly reduced in the patients supplemented with *Aloe vera* compared to placebo controls. A similarly significant benefit was found in glycosylated hemoglobin A1c, triglycerides, total cholesterol, and low-density lipoprotein-cholesterol. *Aloe vera* was superior to placebo in increasing serum high-density lipoprotein-cholesterol. Dr. Zhang said:

Aloe vera has had applications in health and cosmetic products for many centuries, as well as anti-tumor, antioxidant, anti-inflammatory, and laxative properties. It includes over 75 active ingredients that contain enzymes, vitamins, sugars, minerals, lignin, amino acids, and salicylic acid, and most of the constituents appear to be of biological importance in curing diseases.

[Zhang, Y., et al. (2016). Efficacy of *Aloe vera* supplementation on pre-diabetes and early non-treated diabetic patients: A systematic review and meta-analysis of randomized controlled trials. *Nutrients. 2016 Jul; 8 (7): 388.* https://www.ncbi.nlm.nih.gov/pmc/articles/PMC4963864/]

(23) ***Aloe vera*** **decreases fasting blood glucose and improves lipid profiles in type II diabetics and heart disease patients. It reverses angina pectoris symptoms and associated ECG changes.**

Dr. O.P. Agarwal at the 26th Annual Meeting of the American College of Angiology of the International College of Angiology in San Antonio Texas published an article in the August 1985 issue of the journal of *Angiology*. It has been cited by 165 medical articles, which is an impressive number of citations. *Aloe vera* improved fasting blood glucose levels in type II diabetics, improved lipid profiles, and eliminated angina pectoris symptoms and associated ECG changes after three months in heart disease patients. The article describes an extensive study using *Aloe vera* to reverse heart disease.

Five thousand patients with existing angina pectoris and unequivocal ECG changes signifying angina pectoris were studied for five years. Angina pectoris is a heart condition so severe that pain occurs during exercise. Unequivocal ECG changes refer to further objective documentation of the presence of angina pectoris by characteristic electronic measurements of voltages and rhythms produced by the heart.

These patients were treated with *Aloe vera* and a high fiber diet. Total serum cholesterol and triglycerides showed a marked reduction. Diabetics showed a significant decrease in fasting blood glucose.

It is remarkable that during the five years of the *Aloe vera* study involving 5,000 patients with severe heart disease not a single patient died.

Dr. Agarwal says:

Most of the patients started responding from the second week after the therapy was instituted. The improvement was noticed in the form of disappearance of angina pectoris and feeling of well-being. The

ECG changes also started improving, and from 3 months to one year all patients, except 348, had normal ECG tracings even after the treadmill. None of the patients suffered fresh myocardial infarction during the study. The lipid profiles also started improving after three months of the institution of therapy. Out of 5,000 patients, 4,652 patients had normal levels of serum cholesterol ranging from 160-240 mg% and serum triglycerides from 50-90 mg%. Total lipids were from 500-800 mg%, and HDL cholesterol ranged from 50-75 mg%. Out of 3,167 diabetic patients, the blood sugar values, fasting and post-prandial, started coming down to normal levels except in 177 patients, and all the oral hypoglycemic agents had to be withdrawn by the end of two months of therapy. In the entire study, no untoward side effect was noticed, and all the patients were followed for five years from July 1978 to June 1983; all the patients turned up for regular follow-up, and to date, all 5,000 patients are surviving. The diabetic patients, except 177 patients, are on diet control alone, and none have ever complained about any hypoglycemic episode during the study. There is no such study available in the medical literature where such a large number of patients are being followed up for five years, and no Indian plant has ever been tried with such success. So this is a unique study of its own type.

[Agarwal, O.P. (1985). Prevention of atheromatous heart disease. *Angiology. 1985 Aug; 36 (8): 485-92.* https://www.desertharvest.com/physicians/docu ments/DH155.pdf https://bit.ly/angiologystudy https:// pubmed.ncbi.nlm.nih.gov/2864002/]

Aloe vera has benefits for immunity, infections, inflammatory diseases, diabetes, heart disease, aging skin, and age-related diseases.

To summarize again the benefits of *Aloe vera*, we covered the following 23 facts about it.

(1) *Aloe vera* has been used worldwide as a medicinal plant to treat various diseases.

(2) *Aloe vera* activates the immune system against influenza viral infections.

(3) *Aloe vera* restores an immune system damaged by stress.

(4) *Aloe vera* stimulates the immune system's natural killer cell activity against cancer cells.

(5) *Aloe vera* suppresses colon cancer by inhibiting chronic inflammation.

(6) *Aloe vera* cured cancer on the cornea of the eye.

(7) *Aloe vera* has antimicrobial effects against various bacteria, including *Staphylococcus aureus*. These

antimicrobial effects were as strong as those of ofloxacin and ciprofloxacin, potent antibiotics.

(8) *Aloe vera* has antimicrobial effects against antibiotic-resistant strains of *Helicobacter pylori*, the bacteria that can cause stomach ulcers.

(9) *Aloe vera* reduces cigarette smoke-induced lung damage.

(10) *Aloe vera* has anti-inflammatory properties that help gastroesophageal reflux disease.

(11) *Aloe vera* has anti-inflammatory properties that help irritable bowel syndrome.

(12) *Aloe vera* has anti-inflammatory properties that help inflammatory bowel disease.

(13) *Aloe vera* has anti-inflammatory properties that help active ulcerative colitis in 30-47% of patients.

(14) *Aloe vera* has anti-inflammatory properties that help rheumatoid arthritis and the chronic pain of osteoarthritis.

(15) *Aloe vera* has anti-inflammatory properties that help multiple sclerosis.

(16) *Aloe vera* has anti-inflammatory properties that help food allergies and allergic rhinitis.

(17) *Aloe vera* has anti-inflammatory properties that help hypothyroidism in 100% of patients.

(18) *Aloe vera* is equal to chlorhexidine mouthwash

for treating periodontal disease but without the side effects.

(19) *Aloe vera's* polysaccharides derived from the *Aloe vera* gel are safe, non-cytotoxic, and contain no barbaloin, the metabolite responsible for the strong laxative effect of *Aloe vera* latex. It is important to use only the *Aloe vera* gel, not the other two parts of the *Aloe* plant: (1) whole leaf and (2) latex. Beta-mannan™ uses the safe *Aloe vera* gel. An apple is good for you, but that doesn't mean you should eat the bark of its tree. The gel of *Aloe vera* is good for you, but that doesn't mean you should eat the rest of the plant.

(20) *Aloe vera* life-long ingestion in rats prevents age-related diseases and does not cause harmful side effects.

(21) *Aloe vera* significantly improves skin appearance by increasing skin elasticity, hydration, and collagen score in healthy women. This was proven by ultrasound echogenicity. These results suggest that continued *Aloe vera* ingestion contributes to maintaining healthy skin.

(22) *Aloe vera* decreases fasting blood glucose and improves lipid profiles in pre-diabetics.

(23) *Aloe vera* decreases fasting blood glucose and improves lipid profiles in type II diabetics and heart

disease patients. It reverses angina pectoris symptoms and associated ECG changes.

We have seen that *Aloe vera* helps in many areas, particularly enhancing the immune system, fighting viral infections, and decreasing inflammation.

These multiple *Aloe vera* benefits may help explain why patients have found Beta-mannan™ to be effective in eliminating HPV and associated diseases such as cervical dysplasia and warts.

Chapter 25
Comparison of Cervical Dysplasia Treatments

Trichloroacetic acid, or TCA, has no benefit. Beta-carotene, folic acid, and vitamin C may have a slight benefit.

(1) 5-fluorouracil, or 5-FU, has a 50% success when treated for four months, with some side effects.

(2) Indole-3-carbinol has a 44-50% success when treated for three months.

(3) AHCC, or Active Hexose Correlated Compound, has a 44-66% success when treated for 3–7 months, with side effects of nausea, diarrhea, bloating, headache, fatigue, and foot cramps.

(4) **LEEP surgery has a 72.5% success over five years, with the complication of cervical stenosis in 4.3%. Cone biopsy has an 82% success at 27 months, with the complication of cervical stenosis in 10.2%.**

Both procedures have the risk of pre-term delivery due to cervical incompetence.

(5) According to testimonial evidence, Beta-mannan™ has a 95% success when treating cervical dysplasia for three months, with no side effects.

The natural history of the disease would predict a 70% cure rate in 2 years, whereas the evidence shows that Beta-mannan™ has a 95% cure rate in 3 months.

Immunity to HPV is acquired frequently.

Immunity to HPV must specify a particular HPV type - one of the 228 currently identified. If a person tests positive for a particular type or types, but later tests negative for them, then that person has achieved immunity for those particular types, assuming the test result is not a false-negative result.

HPV-negative tests do not rule out an HPV infection because (1) less than 10% of the known 228 HPV types are usually tested, and (2) the tests can yield false-negative results even for the few types tested. Therefore, treatment may be considered if HPV is suspected in the presence of HPV symptoms in the patient or the patient's partner.

Chapter 26
Iodine Benefits for the Immune System and Various Conditions

I odine is a critical mineral for the immune system to prevent and treat infections. Since it has this significant benefit and is deficient in most cultures, increasing iodine intake can help the immune system overcome several things, including HPV infection.

We will cover these 20 facts about iodine and minerals.

(1) Iodine deficiency exists in many cultures including Europe but public awareness of this is poor.

(2) Iodine is a critical mineral for the immune system to prevent and treat thyroid disorders, chronic fatigue, headaches, fibromyalgia, and other infections.

(3) Iodine deficiency leads to fibrocystic breast disease, uterine fibroids, and ovarian cysts. These diseases are likely due to the hyperplastic or extra

tissue growth needed to capture more iodine in an iodine-deficient body.

(4) Iodine is effective in treating fibrocystic breast disease. Iodine supplementation results in 70% improvement for fibrocystic breast disease.

(5) Iodine is beneficial for fibrocystic breast disease and prostate disease. Iodine's high dietary consumption in the Japanese likely explains their low incidence of breast and prostate disease.

(6) Iodine exerts anti-tumor effects against breast, thyroid, and prostate cancer.

(7) The increased prevalence of iodine deficiency in recent decades is likely the cause of an increase in breast cancer in the USA. In contrast, the high iodine consumption in Japanese women is likely responsible for them having an exceptionally low incidence of breast cancer.

(8) A significant increase in iodine deficiency has occurred in the USA since the 1970s. The cause is likely the removal of iodine from bread and its substitution with bromine which further exacerbates iodine deficiency by competing with iodine receptors.

(9) Iodine deficiency explains the increasing incidence of breast cancer in young women in the USA. The high consumption of iodine by specific Asian populations, such as Japanese, correlates with a low

incidence of breast and prostate diseases in those countries.

(10) The recommended dietary intake of iodine in the USA is 100 times too low. People in Japan consume 13.8-200 mg of iodine daily. This amount is 100-1,300 times the USA RDA of only 0.15 mg.

(11) Americans are consuming half as much iodine today compared to 30 years ago. One in seven American women develop breast cancer today compared to one in twenty women 30 years ago, an increase of 300%. The incidence of fibrocystic breast disease was 3% in the 1920s versus 90% today.

(12) The anticancer function of iodine may be one of its most important benefits. Other benefits are suppression of autoimmunity, strengthening the immune system, and protecting against abnormal bacterial growth in the stomach.

(13) Iodine produces a greater sense of well-being, increased energy, clarity of thought, improved skin complexion, and more regular bowel movements. It also increases longevity.

(14) Cancer patients are very iodine deficient.

(15) Iodine deficiency risk is present in over 50% of pregnant women in New York City. This significantly increases the risk of autism and hearing loss in their children.

(16) Iodine deficient children have 6.9-10.2 points lower IQs. Severely iodine deficient children have 12.45 points lower IQs. Iodine deficiency in pregnant mothers can lower the IQs of the children by more than 30 points. Sufficient iodine can increase mental performance in children.

(17) Iodine deficiency is likely a cause of arrhythmias and congestive heart failure.

(18) Selenium supplementation is important when taking iodine because selenium deficiency is common, and selenium is necessary for normal thyroid and immune function.

(19) Magnesium is an important mineral for the immune system but magnesium deficiency is common worldwide.

(20) Calcium is an important mineral for the immune system but calcium deficiency is common worldwide.

Let's take a closer look now at these 20 important facts and the studies that support them.

(1) Iodine deficiency exists in many cultures including Europe but public awareness of this is poor.

Dr. Lucy Kayes at the Centre for Public Health of Queen's University Belfast in Belfast Northern Ireland, and two medical colleagues, published an article in the

July 2022 issue of the *Journal of Nutritional Science* about the current global knowledge of the importance of iodine among women of childbearing age and health-care professionals. Dr. Kayes said:

> Recent population studies in the United Kingdom have found iodine deficiency among schoolgirls, women of childbearing age, and pregnant women. Iodine knowledge is poor among women of child-bearing age in the UK according to four studies using questionnaires and qualitative methods. Globally, there was a similar lack of knowledge.

[Kayes, L., et al. (2022). A review of current knowl-edge about the importance of iodine among women of childbearing age and healthcare professionals. *J Nutr Sci*. 2022 Jul 8; 11: e56. https://pubmed.ncbi.nlm.nih. gov/35836700/]

Dr. Elizabeth A. Miles at the School of Human Development and Health of the Faculty of Medicine of the University of Southampton in Southampton England, and seven medical colleagues, published an article in the March 2022 issue of the *European Journal of Nutrition* about iodine status in pregnant women and infants in Finland. Dr. Miles said:

Of the women studied, 66% had iodine insufficiency at early pregnancy, 70% at late pregnancy, and 59% at three months postpartum. This was also the case in 29% of the three-month-old infants. These observations may have implications for optimal child cognitive development.

[Miles, E.A., et al. (2022). Iodine status in pregnant women and infants in Finland. *Eur J Nutr. 2022 Mar 19.* https://pubmed.ncbi.nlm.nih.gov/35305119/]

Dr. Till Ittermann at the Institute for Community Medicine of the University Medicine Greifswald in Greifswald Germany, and forty-one medical colleagues, published an article in the September 2020 issue of the *Thyroid* journal about iodine deficiency in Europe. Dr. Ittermann said:

We demonstrate that iodine deficiency is still present in Europe, using standardized data from a large number of studies. Adults and pregnant women, particularly, are at risk for iodine deficiency.

[Ittermann, T., et al. (2020). Standardized map of iodine status in Europe. *Thyroid. 2020 Sep; 30 (9): 1346-1354.* https://pubmed.ncbi.nlm.nih.gov/32460688/]

(2) Iodine is a critical mineral for the immune

system to prevent and treat thyroid disorders, chronic fatigue, headaches, fibromyalgia, and other infections.

Dr. Mahmood Y. Bilal at the Clinical Immunology Laboratory of Rosalind Franklin University of Medicine in North Chicago Illinois, and four medical colleagues, published an article in the November 2017 issue of the *Frontiers of Immunology* journal on the value of iodine for immune cells. Dr. Bilal concluded:

Overall, our studies reveal the novel network between human immune cells and thyroid-related molecules and highlight the importance of iodine in regulating the function of human immune cells.

[Bilal, M.Y., et al. (2017). A role for iodide and thyroglobulin in modulating the function of human immune cells. *Front Immunol. 2017 Nov 15; 8: 1573.* https://pubmed.ncbi.nlm.nih.gov/29187856/]

Dr. Guy E. Abraham, a former Professor of Obstetrics, Gynecology, and Endocrinology at the UCLA School of Medicine in Los Angeles California published an article in the October 2004 issue of the *Townsend Letter,* a publication in Port Townsend Washington focusing on Alternative Medicine. Dr. Abraham has received the following honors: the General Diagnostic

Award from the Canadian Association of Clinical Chemists, the Medaille d'Honneur from the University of Liege in Belgium, and the Senior Investigator Award of Pharmacia in Sweden. He co-authored this *Townsend Letter* article with Dr. David Brownstein concerning various aspects of iodine supplementation. Dr. Abraham concluded:

> Our experience has shown that a wide range of disorders has responded to orthoiodo-supplementation, including thyroid disorders, chronic fatigue, headaches, fibromyalgia, and those with infections.

[Abraham, G.E. and Brownstein, D. (2005). *Townsend Letter: A rebuttal of Dr. Gaby's editorial on iodine.* Townsend Letter: Port Townsend, Washington. Retrieved 3 July 2022 https://www.townsendletter.com/Oct2005/gabyrebuttal1005.htm]

Dr. David Brownstein, of the Center for Holistic Medicine in West Bloomfield Michigan, has authored several books about iodine, most notably *Iodine: Why You Need It, Why You Can't Live Without It.* He makes it clear that he has yet to see anything more important for promoting health or optimizing the function of the immune system than iodine.

[Brownstein, D. (2009). *Iodine: Why You Need It,*

Why You Can't Live Without It (4th Edition). West Bloomfield, Michigan: Medical Alternatives Press.]

(3) Iodine deficiency leads to fibrocystic breast disease, uterine fibroids, and ovarian cysts. These diseases are likely due to the hyperplastic or extra tissue growth needed to capture more iodine in an iodine-deficient body.

Dr. Saeed Kagar and four medical colleagues at the Department of General Surgery of Shahid Sadoughi University of Medical Sciences in Yazd Iran published an article in the March 2017 issue of the *Asian Pacific Journal of Cancer Prevention*. Dr. Kagar said:

> It is proven that iodine deficiency can lead to fibro-cystic breast disease and/or ovarian cysts. Iodine can similarly reduce uterine fibroids, and one of the first conventional medical treatments for severe fibroids was to paint the uterus with iodine.

[Kargar, S., et al. (2017). Urinary iodine concentrations in cancer patients. *Asian Pac J Cancer Prev. 2017 Mar 1; 18 (3): 819-821.* https://www.ncbi.nlm.nih.gov/pmc/articles/PMC5464505/]

(4) Iodine is effective in treating fibrocystic breast disease. Iodine supplementation results in 70% improvement for fibrocystic breast disease.

Dr. W.R. Ghent and three medical colleagues at the Department of Surgery of Queen's University in Kingston Ontario Canada published an article in the October 1993 issue of the *Canadian Journal of Surgery* about using iodine to treat fibrocystic disease of the breast. Dr. Ghent found that 70% of women improved their fibrocystic breast disease with iodine replacement therapy.

[Ghent, W.R., et al. (1993). Iodine replacement in fibrocystic disease of the breast. *Can J Surg. 1993 Oct; 36 (5):* 453-60. https://pubmed.ncbi.nlm.nih.gov/8221402/]

Dr. Bernard A. Eskin at the Department of Obstetrics and Gynecology of the Medical College of Pennsylvania in Philadelphia Pennsylvania published an article in the August 1983 issue of the *Biological Trace Element Research* journal about iodine and breast cancer. Dr. Eskin concluded:

In many controlled studies, iodine has been established as a requirement for breast tissue normalcy since deficiency of the element results in histopathology consistent with dysplasia and atypia in rodents. Clinically severe hyperplasia and fibrocystic disease are seen in the breasts of women who have low iodine levels. These precancerous lesions result in a high-risk state as well as persistent sympto-matology in women. Iodine replacement therapy has been shown to be efficacious in reducing these conditions in clinical trials.

[Eskin, B.A. (1983). Iodine and breast cancer: 1982 update. *Biol Trace Elem Res. 1983 Aug; 5 (4-5): 399-412,* https://pubmed.ncbi.nlm.nih.gov/24263577/]

(5) Iodine is beneficial for fibrocystic breast disease and prostate disease. Iodine's high dietary consumption in the Japanese likely explains their low incidence of breast and prostate disease.

Dr. Carmen Aceves and two medical colleagues at the Institute of Neurobiology of the National Autonomous University of Mexico in Juriquilla Mexico published an article in the August 2013 issue of the *Thyroid* journal about various benefits of iodine. Dr. Aceves said:

Several tissues share with the thyroid gland the capacity to actively accumulate iodine; these include the salivary glands, gastric mucosa, lactating mammary gland, the choroid plexus, ciliary body of the eye, lacrimal gland, thymus, skin, placenta, ovary, uterus, prostate, and pancreas, and they may either maintain or lose this ability under pathological conditions. Similarly, I2 treatment (3–6 mg/day) of patients with benign breast disease is accompanied by a significant bilateral reduction in breast size and remission of disease symptoms. Moreover, similar benefits have been found in benign prostatic hyperplasia and in human patients with early benign prostatic hyperplasia (stages I and II), where an 8-month Lugol's (5 mg/day) supplement was accompanied by diminished symptoms and prostate-specific antigen values, and an increased urine flow rate. All these data agree with epidemiological reports showing a direct association in the Japanese population between the low incidence of breast and prostate pathologies and the moderately high dietary intake of iodine. Seaweeds, which are widely consumed in Asian countries, contain high quantities of iodine in several chemical forms; the average iodine consumption in the Japanese population is 1,200–5,280 mcg/day versus 166 and 209 mcg/day in the United Kingdom and the United States, respectively.

[Aceves, C., et al. (2013). The extrathyronine actions of iodine as antioxidant, apoptotic, and differentiation factor in various tissues. *Thyroid. 2013 Aug; 23 (8): 938–946.* https://www.ncbi.nlm.nih.gov/pmc/articles/PMC3752513/]

(6) Iodine exerts anti-tumor effects against breast, thyroid, and prostate cancer.

Dr. Nuri Aranda and four medical colleagues at the Departamento de Neurobiología Celular y Molecular of the Universidad Nacional Autónoma de México in Querétaro Mexico published an article in the January 2013 issue of the *Prostate* journal concerning the anti-tumor effects of iodine. Dr. Aranda said regarding iodine's effect on apoptosis, or cell death, of cancer cells:

> Evidence indicates that iodine per se could be implicated in the physiology of several organs that can internalize it. In thyroid and breast cancer, iodine treatments inhibit cell proliferation and induce apoptosis. Here, we determined the uptake of iodide and iodine, as well as the anti-proliferative and apoptotic effects of 6-iodolactone and both forms of iodine in human prostate cells lines. Normal and cancerous prostate cells can take up iodine, and depending on the chemical form, it exerts anti-proliferative and apoptotic effects both in vitro and in vivo.

[Aranda, N., et al. (2013). Uptake and anti-tumoral effects of iodine and 6-iodolactone in differentiated and undifferentiated human prostate cancer cell lines.

Prostate. 2013 Jan; 73 (1): 31-41. https://pubmed.ncbi. nlm.nih.gov/22576883/]

(7) The increased prevalence of iodine deficiency in recent decades is likely the cause of an increase in breast cancer in the USA. In contrast, the high iodine consumption in Japanese women is likely responsible for them having an exceptionally low incidence of breast cancer.

Dr. Jay Rappaport at the Department of Neuroscience of Lewis Katz School of Medicine of Temple University in Philadelphia Pennsylvania published an article in the January 2017 issue of the *Journal of Cancer*. He explained that the increased incidence of breast cancer in the USA is a result of the low dietary intake of iodine. Dr. Rappaport said:

Iodine deficiency has been proposed to play a causative role in the development of breast cancer. Dietary iodine has also been previously proposed to play a protective role in breast cancer, to a large degree based on the increased iodine consumption of dietary iodine in Japanese women, having an exceptionally low incidence of breast cancer. Furthermore, emigration of Japanese women adopting a western diet is associated with higher breast cancer rates. Iodine is taken up by the sodium/iodide symporter in the breast, and its role is important in promoting the development of normal versus neoplastic breast tissue development. In animal models of breast cancer, iodine in supplement or seaweed form has demonstrated beneficial effects in suppressing breast cancer cell and tumor growth. The mechanism of action of iodine's anticancer effect may be complex, and roles as an antioxidant, promoting differentiation and apoptosis related to breast cancer have been proposed.

Dr. Rappaport also stated about a deficiency of iodine:

Increased iodine demand in women is likely due to the increased uptake of iodine in breast tissue, in addition to the thyroid gland, where iodine plays a role in the development and maintenance of healthy breast tissue (expanding after puberty) and in breast remodeling during lactation, and pregnancy. Young women and, to a greater extent, pregnant women have lower urinary iodine levels than men of similar age. According to the CDC's 2012 Second National Report of Biochemical Indicators of Diet and Nutrition in the USA Population, women of childbearing age exhibited the lowest urinary iodine levels of any age group.

Iodine deficiency is associated with fibrocystic breast disease, which can be effectively treated or prevented with iodine supplementation. Fibrocystic breast disease affects at least 50% of women of childbearing age and is associated with an increased risk of developing breast cancer.

(8) A significant increase in iodine deficiency has occurred in the USA since the 1970s. The cause is likely the removal of iodine from bread and its substitution with bromine which further exacerbates iodine deficiency by competing with iodine receptors.

Dr. Rappaport outlines the development of iodine deficiency that has occurred in recent years in the USA:

Comparisons of the National Health and Nutrition Examination Surveys showed a significant decrease in urinary iodine levels in the overall population during the period 1988-1994 as compared to the period 1971-1974. Accordingly, the percentage of total persons with iodine deficiency increased from 2.6% during the period 1971-1974, to 14.5% in 1988-1994, representing a 5.6-fold increase. Females showed a higher frequency of iodine deficiency than males (15.1% versus 8.1%). For young women of childbearing age, age 15-44, there was a 3.8-fold increase in iodine insufficiency, with a 6.9-fold increase in the number of pregnant women also fitting this definition.

Dr. Rappaport said:

In addition to the potential risk for breast cancer, even mild iodine insufficiency appears to correlate with neurocognitive impairments in children. Thus, iodine insufficiency represents a major health issue for women of childbearing age as well as developing fetuses. The observed drop in urinary iodine in young women as well as in the general population, since the 1970s, is presumably due to the removal of iodine from bread and substitution with bromine as flour conditioner during this period, due in large part to previous concerns about excess iodine as well as the preferences of commercial bakers for brominated flour. Bromine, a suspected carcinogen, may further exacerbate iodine insufficiency since bromine competes for iodine uptake by the thyroid gland and potentially other tissues (i.e., the breast). The annual increase in distant breast cancer diagnosis since the mid-1970s may reflect the time of exposure to decreased iodine and increased dietary bromine.

(9) Iodine deficiency explains the increasing incidence of breast cancer in young women in the USA. The high consumption of iodine by specific Asian populations, such as Japanese, correlates with a low incidence of breast and prostate diseases in those countries.

Dr. Rappaport says:

In conclusion, dietary iodine insufficiency represents a plausible explanation for the increasing incidence of breast cancer in young women with distant metastasis. In view of the established reduction in iodine levels in USA women of childbearing age since the mid-70s, this group would be most vulnerable to increased breast cancer risk. Based on the importance of iodine in thyroid and breast health, fetal brain development, and deficits in nutritional trends among younger women, iodine testing and management may be considered a potentially important aspect for clinical practice.

[Rappaport, J. (2017). Changes in dietary iodine explains increasing incidence of breast cancer with distant involvement in young women. *J Cancer. 2017; 8 (2): 174–177.* https://www.ncbi.nlm.nih.gov/pmc/articles/PMC5327366/]

Dr. Brenda Anguiano and Dr. Carmen Aceves at the Institute of Neurobiology of the National Autonomous University of Mexico in Juriquilla Mexico published an article in the 2011 issue of the *Current Chemical Biology* journal concerning iodine, breast, and prostate disease. Dr. Anguiano said:

A robust body of information supports the notion that moderately high concentrations of iodine may reduce pathologies in several tissues that concentrate iodine. This paper reviews evidence showing iodine to be an antioxidant and apoptotic agent that may contribute to the differentiation of normal mammary and prostate glands. In animal and human studies, molecular iodine supplements suppress the development and size of both benign and malignant neoplasias in these glands. Iodine, in addition to its incorporation into thyroid hormones, is bound to anti-proliferative iodolipids called iodolactones, which may play a role in controlling proliferative pathologies in mammary and prostate glands. These studies are in line with data demonstrating that the high consumption of iodine by certain Asian populations, such as in Japan, correlates with a low incidence of benign and cancerous breast and prostate diseases. Based on our data, we proposed that an I2 supplement should be considered as an adjuvant in the treatment of pathologies in breast and prostate.

[Anguiano, B., et al. (2011). Iodine in mammary and prostate pathologies. *Current Chemical Biology, Volume 5, Number 3, 2011, pp. 177-182 (6)*. https://www.ingenta connect.com/content/ben/ccb/2011/00000005/00000003/art00005]

(10) The recommended dietary intake of iodine in the USA is 100 times too low. People in Japan consume 13.8-200 mg of iodine daily. This amount is 100-1,300 times the USA RDA of only 0.15 mg.

Dr. Donald W. Miller, Jr. at the Division of Cardio-thoracic Surgery of the University of Washington School of Medicine in Seattle Washington published an article in the 2006 issue of the *Journal of American Physicians and Surgeons*. It concerned the benefits of iodine for extra-thyroidal tissues, which means tissues other than the thyroid gland. Dr. Miller said:

In addition to being an essential element in thyroid hormones, iodine has many biological functions. The recommended dietary intake of 100–150 mcg is perhaps 100 times too low. Potential benefits of higher amounts include enhancement of immune function and reducing the incidence of breast cancer.

Dr. Miller emphasized:

In 1964, the Nutrition Section of Japan's Bureau of Public Health found that people in Japan consumed a daily average of 4.5 g of seaweed with a measured iodine content of 3.1 mg/g, or 13.8 mg of iodine. According to bureau officials, seaweed consumption in Japan is now 14.5 g, providing 45 mg of iodine. Studies measuring urine concentration of iodine confirm that the Japanese consume iodine in milligram amounts. And researchers have determined that residents on the coast of Hokkaido eat a quantity of seaweed sufficient to provide a daily iodine intake of 200 mg/day. Saltwater fish and shellfish contain iodine, but one would have to eat 15–25 pounds of fish to get 13 mg of iodine.

(11) Americans are consuming half as much iodine today compared to 30 years ago. One in seven American women develop breast cancer today compared to one in twenty women 30 years ago, an increase of 300%. The incidence of fibrocystic breast disease was 3% in the 1920s versus 90% today.

Moreover, Dr. Miller explained regarding iodine intake in Japan compared to the USA:

The average daily intake of iodine in the USA is 240 mcg, well within the range that the International Council for the Control of Iodine Deficiency Disorders defines as an optimal iodine intake, 150-299 mcg/day. Though considered iodine sufficient, this amount, 0.24 mg, is a small fraction of that consumed in Japan. Also, this is half the amount of iodine Americans consumed 30 years ago when iodine was used more widely in the dairy industry and as a dough conditioner in making bread. Now it is only added to table salt, and 45 percent of American households buy salt without iodine. And over the last 25 years those who do use iodized table salt have decreased their consumption of it by 65 percent. As a result, 15 percent of the USA adult female population, one in seven, suffers from iodine deficiency, as reflected in a urinary iodine concentration of less than 50 mcg/L. One in seven American women now also develop breast cancer during their lifetime (30 years ago it was 1 in 20).

Regarding fibrocystic breast disease, Dr. Miller points out:

The incidence of fibrocystic breast disease in American women was 3 percent in the 1920s. Today, 90 percent of women have this disorder, manifested by epithelial hyperplasia, apocrine gland metaplasia, fluid-filled cysts, and fibrosis. Six million American women with fibrocystic breast disease have moderate to severe breast pain and tenderness that lasts more than six days during the menstrual cycle.

(12) The anticancer function of iodine may be one of its most important benefits. Other benefits are suppression of autoimmunity, strengthening the immune system, and protecting against abnormal bacterial growth in the stomach.

Regarding apoptosis, Dr. Miller said:

Iodine induces apoptosis. This process of programmed cell death is essential to growth and development and for destroying cells that represent a threat to the integrity of the organism, like cancer cells and cells infected with viruses. It is hypothe-sized that anticancer function may well prove to be iodine's most important extra-thyroidal benefit. Epidemiological studies show that a high intake of iodine is associated with a low incidence of breast cancer and a low intake with a high incidence of breast cancer.

Furthermore, Dr. Miller states regarding iodine's benefits:

> It removes toxic chemicals and biological toxins; suppresses autoimmunity; strengthens the T-cell adaptive immune system; and protects against abnormal growth of bacteria in the stomach, *Helicobacter pylori* in particular.

(13) Iodine produces a greater sense of well-being, increased energy, clarity of thought, improved skin complexion, and more regular bowel movements. It also increases longevity.

Referring to the recommendations of Dr. Guy Abraham, a former Professor of Obstetrics, Gynecology, and Endocrinology at the UCLA School of Medicine in Los Angeles California, Dr. Miller says:

> Consumption of iodine in milligram doses should be coupled with a complete nutritional program that includes, in particular, adequate amounts of selenium, magnesium, and omega-3 fatty acids. So done, Dr. Abraham believes that taking 12.5 mg/day of iodine is *the simplest, safest, most effective, and least expensive way* to help solve many medical problems. Many subjective benefits have been claimed for milligram-dose

iodine: a greater sense of well-being, increased energy, and a lifting of brain fog. Patients also report that they feel warmer in cold environments, need somewhat less sleep, have improved skin complexion, and have more regular bowel movements. These are in addition to the improvements in fibrocystic disease of the breast, and a possibly reduced incidence of breast cancer noted above.

[Miller, D.W. (2006). Extra-thyroidal benefits of iodine. *Journal of American Physicians and Surgeons, Volume 11, Number 4, Winter 2006.* https://www.jpands. org/jpands1104.htm   https://www.ign.org/cm_data/ 2006_Miller_Extrathyroidal_Benefits_of_Iodine.pdf]

Dr. Johannes Riis at the Department of Geriatric Medicine of Aalborg University Hospital in Aalborg Denmark, and nine medical colleagues, published an article in the February 2021 issue of the *British Journal of Nutrition* describing long-term iodine nutrition as being associated with longevity. Dr. Riis concluded:

Residing in iodine-replete Skagen was associated with increased longevity. This indicates that long-term residency in an iodine-replete environment may be associated with increased longevity compared with residency in an iodine-deficient environment.

[Riis, J., et al. (2021). Long-term iodine nutrition is associated with longevity in older adults: a 20 years' follow-up of the Randers-Skagen study. *Br J Nutr. 2021 Feb 14; 125 (3): 260-265.* https://pubmed.ncbi.nlm.nih.gov/32378500/]

(14) Cancer patients are very iodine deficient.

Dr. Saeed Kagar and four medical colleagues at the Department of General Surgery of Shahid Sadoughi University of Medical Sciences in Yazd Iran published an article in the March 2017 issue of the *Asian Pacific Journal of Cancer Prevention* about iodine deficiencies in cancer patients. Dr. Kagar said:

It has been suggested that the incidence of some cancers, especially examples in the breast and stomach, may be influenced by the iodine intake. Therefore, we have conducted the present assessment of iodine status in Iranian patients diagnosed with a malignancy. Iranian cancer patients were seriously iodine deficient.

[Kargar, S., et al. (2017). Urinary iodine concentrations in cancer patients. *Asian Pac J Cancer Prev. 2017 Mar 1; 18 (3): 819-821.* https://www.ncbi.nlm.nih.gov/pmc/articles/PMC5464505/]

(15) Iodine deficiency risk is present in over 50%

of pregnant women in New York City. This significantly increases the risk of autism and hearing loss in their children.

Dr. Rachel Pessah-Pollack and three medical colleagues at the Division of Endocrinology of Mount Sinai Medical Center in New York New York published an article in the January 2014 issue of *Journal of Women's Health*. They discussed iodine supplementation during pregnancy. Dr. Pessah-Pollack concluded:

Pregnant women are at increased risk for iodine deficiency, which may induce thyroid insufficiency and have damaging effects not only on the mother but also on the fetus. Overall, more than one out of two pregnant women in New York City were at risk for iodine deficiency. New York City pregnant women were significantly less prone to iodine deficiency when provided with iodine supplementation. Nevertheless, when spot urine iodine levels were used to estimate iodine sufficiency, more than 20% of supplemented women were still at risk for iodine deficiency, according to WHO guidelines, suggesting that current supplementation practices remain insufficient.

[Pessah-Pollack, R., et al. (2014). Apparent insufficiency of iodine supplementation in pregnancy. *J*

Womens Health (Larchmt). 2014 Jan; 23 (1): 51-6. https://pubmed.ncbi.nlm.nih.gov/24117002/]

Dr. Rasha T. Hamza and two medical colleagues at the Department of Pediatrics of the Faculty of Medicine of Ain Shams University in Cairo Egypt published an article in the October 2013 issue of *Archives of Medical Research* journal on the relationship of iodine deficiency to autism. Dr. Hamza determined that iodine deficiency is prevalent in Egyptian autistic children and in their mothers and was directly related to disease severity. Dr. Hamza said:

> Fifty autistic children and their mothers were studied in comparison to 50 controls. Of autistic children and their mothers, 54% and 58%, respectively, were iodine deficient. None of the control children or their mothers was iodine deficient.

[Hamza, R.T., et al. (2013). Iodine deficiency in Egyptian autistic children and their mothers: relation to disease severity. *Arch Med Res. 2013 Oct; 44 (7): 555-61.* https://pubmed.ncbi.nlm.nih.gov/24120386/]

Dr. P. Valeix and four medical colleagues at the Institut Scientifique et Technique de la Nutrition in Paris France published an article in the January 1999 issue of the *European Journal of Clinical Nutrition* on iodine status and the hearing capacity in 1,222 children. Dr. Valeix found that hearing loss was more severe among children with iodine deficiency. Dr. Valeix said: "Hearing loss at 4000 Hz and average hearing impairment at speech frequencies (500, 1000, and 2000 Hz) were more severe among children at risk of mild to moderate iodine deficiency."

[Valeix, P., et al. (1994). Relationship between urinary iodine concentration and hearing capacity in children. *Eur J Clin Nutr. 1994 Jan; 48 (1): 54-9.* https://pubmed.ncbi.nlm.nih.gov/8200329/]

(16) Iodine deficient children have 6.9-10.2 points lower IQs. Severely iodine deficient children have 12.45 points lower IQs. Iodine deficiency in pregnant mothers can lower the IQs of the children by more than 30 points. Sufficient iodine can increase mental performance in children.

Dr. Karim Bougma and three medical colleagues at the School of Dietetics and Human Nutrition of McGill University in Quebec Canada published an article in the April 2013 issue of the *Nutrients* journal that examined the relationship between iodine and mental development of children 5 years old and under. Dr. Bougma found that iodine-deficient children had 6.9-10.2 points lower IQs. Dr. Bougma said: "Iodine deficiency had a substantial impact on mental development."

[Bougma, K., et al. (2013). Iodine and mental development of children 5 years old and under: a systematic review and meta-analysis. *Nutrients. 2013 Apr 22; 5 (4): 1384-416.* https://pubmed.ncbi.nlm.nih.gov/23609774/]

Dr. Ming Qian and five medical colleagues at the Institute of Endocrinology of the Tianjin Medical University in Tianjin China published an article in the 2005 issue of the *Asia Pacific Journal of Clinical Nutrition* about the effects of iodine on the intelligence of children. Thirty-seven studies with a total of 12,291 children were analyzed. The intelligence damage of children exposed to severe iodine deficiency was profound, demonstrated by a 12.45 IQ points loss. Dr. Qian said: "Iodine supplementation before and during pregnancy to women living in severe iodine-deficient areas could prevent their children from intelligence deficit."

[Qian, M., et al. (2005). The effects of iodine on intelligence in children: a meta-analysis of studies conducted in China. *Asia Pac J Clin Nutr. 2005; 14 (1): 32-42.* https://pubmed.ncbi.nlm.nih.gov/15734706/]

Dr. S.C. Boyages and five medical colleagues at the Department of Medicine of the University of Sydney in New South Wales Australia published an article in the June 1989 issue of the *Medical Journal of Australia* about

intellectual impairment resulting from iodine deficiency. Dr. Boyages concluded:

> In urban school children who were aged seven to 14
> years, a normal range of measured intelligence was
> found to be 107. In villagers who were born during the
> period of severe iodine deficiency, 72% had an intelli-
> gence-quotient score of less than 70. In the iodine-
> deficient village, lower intelligence-quotient scores
> showed a relationship with the detection by audiom-
> etry of nerve deafness and with the presence of
> abnormal neurological signs. The latter included spas-
> ticity and pyramidal signs which were a similar
> pattern to the neurological deficits that have been
> demonstrated in overt neurological cretins.

[Boyages, S.C., et al. (1989). Iodine deficiency
impairs intellectual and neuromotor development in
apparently normal persons. A study of rural inhabitants
of north-central China. *Med J Aust. 1989 Jun 19; 150 (12):
676-82.* https://pubmed.ncbi.nlm.nih.gov/2733614/]

Dr. Tina Van Den Briel and five medical colleagues
at the Division of Human Nutrition and Epidemiology
of Wageningen University in Wageningen Netherlands
published an article in the November 2000 issue of the
American Journal of Clinical Nutrition. This encouraging

article showed that the mental status of children improved with iodine supplementation. Dr. Van Den Briel said:

An adequate iodine supply in utero and shortly after birth is known to be crucial to an individual's physical and mental development. The aim of this study was to examine the effect of an improvement in iodine status on mental and psychomotor performance of school children who were moderately to severely iodine deficient. Children with increased urinary iodine concentrations had a significantly greater increase in performance on the combination of mental tests than did the group with no change in urinary iodine concentrations. These findings suggest a catch-up effect in terms of mental performance.

[Van Den Briel, T., et al. (2000). Improved iodine status is associated with improved mental performance of school children in Benin. *Am J Clin Nutr. 2000 Nov; 72 (5): 1179-85.* https://pubmed.ncbi.nlm.nih.gov/11063446/]

(17) Iodine deficiency is likely a cause of arrhythmias and congestive heart failure.

Dr. I. Molnar at the Department of Internal Medicine of Kenézy County and Teaching Hospital in

Debrecen Hungary, and two medical colleagues, published an article in the February 2007 issue of the journal of *Orvosi Hetilap* concerning iodine deficiency in cardiovascular diseases. Dr. Molnar said: "The most decreased urine iodine concentration was detected in the subgroups with arrhythmia and congestive heart failure."

[Molnar, I., et al. (1998). Iodine deficiency in cardiovascular diseases. *Orv Hetil. 1998 Aug 30; 139 (35): 2071-3.* https://pubmed.ncbi.nlm.nih.gov/9755626/]

(18) Selenium supplementation is important when taking iodine because selenium deficiency is common, and selenium is necessary for normal thyroid and immune function.

Dr. J.R. Arthur and two medical colleagues at the Division of Micronutrient and Lipid Metabolism of Rowett Research Institute in Aberdeen Scotland published an article in the June 1999 issue of the journal of *Nutrition Research Reviews* about the importance of adequate intake of selenium in iodine deficiency. Dr. Arthur said:

> Since selenium has an essential role in thyroid hormone metabolism, it has the potential to play a major part in the outcome of iodine deficiency. These effects of selenium derive from two aspects of its

biological function. First, three selenium-containing deiodinases regulate the synthesis and degradation of the biologically active thyroid hormone, T3. Second, selenoperoxidases and possibly thioredoxin reductase protect the thyroid gland from H2O2 produced during the synthesis of thyroid hormones. The mechanisms whereby selenium deficiency exacerbates the hypothyroidism due to iodine deficiency have been elucidated in animals. The protection of the thyroid gland from H2O2 and the regulation of tissue T3 levels are the functions of selenium that are most likely to underlie the interactions of selenium and iodine.

[Arthur, J.R., et al. (1999). The interactions between selenium and iodine deficiencies in man and animals. *Nutr Res Rev. 1999 Jun; 12 (1): 55-73.* https://pubmed. ncbi.nlm.nih.gov/19087446/]

Dr. Lutz Schomburg and a medical colleague at the Institute of Experimental Endocrinology of Charity University Medical School in Berlin Germany published an article in the November 2008 issue of the *Molecular Nutrition and Food Research* journal about the importance of selenium and iodine. Dr. Schomburg said:

The trace elements iodine and selenium are essential for thyroid gland functioning and thyroid hormone biosynthesis and metabolism. While iodine is needed as the eponymous constituent of the two major thyroid hormones T3 and T4, selenium is essential for the biosynthesis and function of a small number of selenocysteine-containing selenoproteins implicated in thyroid hormone metabolism and gland function. The selenium-dependent iodothyronine deiodinases control thyroid hormone turnover, while both intra-cellular and secreted selenium-dependent glutathione peroxidases are implicated in gland protection. Recently, a number of clinical supplemen-tation trials have indicated positive effects of increasing the selenium status of the participants in a variety of pathologies. These findings enforce the notion that many people might profit from improving their selenium status, both as a means to reduce the individual health risk as well as to balance a selenium deficiency which often develops during the course of illness. The effects of selenium appear to be exerted via multiple mechanisms that impact most pronounced on the endocrine and the immune systems.

[Schomburg, L., et al. (2008). On the importance of selenium and iodine metabolism for thyroid hormone biosynthesis and human health. *Mol Nutr Food Res.*

2008 Nov; 52 (11): 1235-46. https://pubmed.ncbi.nlm.
nih.gov/18686295/]

Dr. J. Kvicala and a medical colleague at the Institute of Endocrinology in Prague Czech Republic published an article in the *Central European Journal of Public Health* about the effect of iodine and selenium on thyroid function. Dr. Kvicala said:

> Essential trace element selenium has a fundamental importance to the cell and body metabolism regulation by thyroid hormones. Especially dangerous are concomitant deficiencies of both key elements for thyroid hormone metabolism - iodine and selenium - from the point of thyroid hormone regulative functions.

[Kvicala, J., et al. (2003). Effect of iodine and selenium upon thyroid function. *Cent Eur J Public Health.* *2003 Jun; 11 (2): 107-13.* https://pubmed.ncbi.nlm.nih.
gov/12884559/]

Dr. S.A. Cann and two medical colleagues at the Special Development Laboratory of Royal Jubilee Hospital in Victoria British Columbia Canada published an article in the February 2000 issue of *Cancer Causes and Control* journal about iodine and selenium. Dr. Cann said:

In this paper we examine some of the evidence linking iodine and selenium to breast cancer development. Seaweed is a popular dietary component in Japan and a rich source of both of these essential elements. We hypothesize that this dietary preference may be associated with the low incidence of benign and malignant breast disease in Japanese women. In animal and human studies, iodine administration has been shown to cause regression of both iodine-deficient goiter and benign pathological breast tissue. Iodine, in addition to its incorporation into thyroid hormones, is organified into anti-proliferative iodolipids in the thyroid; such compounds may also play a role in the proliferative control of extra-thyroidal tissues. Selenium acts synergistically with iodine. All three mono-deiodinase enzymes are selenium-dependent and are involved in thyroid hormone regulation. In this way selenium status may affect both thyroid hormone homeostasis and iodine availability.

[Cann, S.A., et al. (2000). Hypothesis: iodine, selenium and the development of breast cancer. *Cancer Causes Control. 2000 Feb; 11 (2): 121-7.* https://pubmed. ncbi.nlm.nih.gov/10710195/]

Dr. Francesca Gorini at the Institute of Clinical

Physiology National Research Council in Pisa Italy, and three medical colleagues, published an article in the November 2021 issue of the journal of *Molecules of Basel Switzerland* about selenium. Dr. Gorini said:

> Selenium, a micro-element essential for life, is critical for homeostasis of several critical functions, such as those related to immune-endocrine function. In particular, selenium is critical for the function of the thyroid, and it is particularly abundant in this gland. Unfortunately, selenium deficiency is a very common condition worldwide. Supplementation is possible, but as selenium has a narrow safety level, toxic levels are close to those normally required for a correct need.

[Gorini, F., et al. (2021). Selenium: An element of life essential for thyroid function. *Molecules. 2021 Nov 23; 26 (23): 7084.* https://pubmed.ncbi.nlm.nih.gov/34885664/]

Dr. Marek Kieliszek at the Faculty of Food Sciences of the Department of Biotechnology of Warsaw University of Life Sciences in Warsaw Poland published an article in the April 2019 issue of the *Molecules* journal about selenium daily dosage requirements. Dr. Kieliszek said:

Daily doses of this element in the range of 100–200 mcg lead to the reduction of genetic damage. In addition, it is considered that selenium may be an important factor in the prevention of cancer development. Selenium consumption at the level of 200 mcg per day leads to the increased formation of cytotoxic T cells and natural killer cells. The results of studies conducted in the UK have shown that consumption of 100 mcg of selenium a day relieves the symptoms of depression and anxiety. The dose that does not show any adverse effect for adults is estimated at 800 mcg Se/day, whereas a dose that causes the onset of toxicity ranges from 1540-1600 mcg Se/day. The content of selenium in food products in a given geographical region is proportional to its amount in the soil present in that region. Therefore, the amount of this element in food differs for similar products from particular regions of the world. In the United States, it slightly exceeds 90 mcg per day. In some European countries, the intake of this element is below the recommended value (~30 mcg/day).

[Kieliszek, M. (2019). Selenium–fascinating microelement, properties and sources in food. *Molecules. 2019 Apr; 24 (7): 1298.* https://www.ncbi.nlm.nih.gov/pmc/articles/PMC6480557/]

(19) Magnesium is an important mineral for the immune system but magnesium deficiency is common worldwide.

Dr. Kunling Wang at the Department of Endocrinology and Metabolism of Tianjin Medical University in Tianjin China, and thirteen medical colleagues, published an article in the 2018 issue of the *Scientific Reports* journal about magnesium deficiency. Dr. Wang said:

Epidemiological surveys show that magnesium deficiency exists in many regions worldwide. According to data from the National Health and Nutrition Examination (2001–2010) in the United States, the magnesium intakes of only 18.8% of male participants and 24.8% of female participants met the recommended dietary allowance. Magnesium is closely related to the immune system; in vitro experiments have showed that intracellular free magnesium ions are an important second messenger in the immune activation of T lymphocytes and B lymphocytes, and magnesium channels and transport proteins play an important role in normal immune function.

[Wang, K., et al. (2018). Severely low serum magnesium is associated with increased risks of positive anti-thyroglobulin antibody and hypothyroidism: A cross-sectional study. *Sci Rep. 2018; 8: 9904.* https://www.ncbi.nlm.nih.gov/pmc/articles/PMC6028657/]

Dr. James J. DiNicolantonio at the Department of Preventive Cardiology of Saint Luke's Mid America Heart Institute in Kansas City Missouri, and two medical colleagues, published an article in the January 2018 issue of the *Open Heart* journal about subclinical magnesium deficiency. Dr. DiNicolantonio said:

> Because serum magnesium does not reflect intracellular magnesium, the latter making up more than 99% of total body magnesium, most cases of magnesium deficiency are undiagnosed. The vast majority of people in modern societies are at risk for magnesium deficiency. Importantly, subclinical magnesium deficiency does not manifest as clinically apparent symptoms and thus is not easily recognized by the clinician. Despite this fact, subclinical magnesium deficiency likely leads to hypertension, arrhythmias, arterial calcifications, atherosclerosis, heart failure and an increased risk for thrombosis. This suggests that subclinical magnesium deficiency is a principal, yet under-recognized, driver of cardiovascular disease. A greater public health effort is needed to inform both

the patient and clinician about the prevalence, harms and diagnosis of subclinical magnesium deficiency.

[DiNicolantonio, J.J., et al. (2018). Subclinical magnesium deficiency: a principal driver of cardiovascular disease and a public health crisis. *Open Heart. 2018; 5 (1): e000668.* https://www.ncbi.nlm.nih.gov/pmc/articles/PMC5786912/]

(20) Calcium is an important mineral for the immune system but calcium deficiency is common worldwide.

Dr. Julie Shlisky at the New York Academy of Sciences in New York New York and fourteen medical colleagues published an article in the June 2022 issue of the *Annals of the New York Academy of Sciences* journal about calcium deficiency. Dr. Shlisky said:

Dietary calcium deficiency is considered to be widespread globally, with published estimates suggesting that approximately half of the world's population has inadequate access to dietary calcium. Calcium is essential for bone health, but inadequate intakes have also been linked to other health outcomes, including pregnancy complications, cancers, and cardiovascular disease.

[Shlisky, J., et al. (2022). Calcium deficiency world-wide: prevalence of inadequate intakes and associated health outcomes. *Ann N Y Acad Sci. 2022 Jun; 1512 (1): 10-28.* https://pubmed.ncbi.nlm.nih.gov/35247225/]

Dr. Mark A. Plantz at Northwestern University in Evanston Illinois and a medical colleague published an article in the May 2022 issue of *Stat Pearls* about dietary calcium. Dr. Plantz said:

> The most recent daily value for calcium is 1,300 mg for adults and children older than four years of age. Sufficient calcium intake is achievable from a well-balanced diet, but many patients do not eat a well-balanced diet.

[Plantz, M.A., et al. (2022). Dietary Calcium. Treasure Island, Florida: *StatPearls Publishing. May 22, 2022.* https://www.ncbi.nlm.nih.gov/books/NBK549792/]

Iodine is a critical mineral for the immune system to prevent and treat infections. Since it has this significant benefit and is deficient in most cultures, increasing iodine intake can help the immune system function effectively, including against HPV infection.

To summarize again the benefits of iodine and

minerals, we covered the following 20 facts about them.

(1) Iodine deficiency exists in many cultures including Europe but public awareness of this is poor.

(2) Iodine is a critical mineral for the immune system to prevent and treat thyroid disorders, chronic fatigue, headaches, fibromyalgia, and other infections.

(3) Iodine deficiency leads to fibrocystic breast disease, uterine fibroids, and ovarian cysts. These diseases are likely due to the hyperplastic or extra tissue growth needed to capture more iodine in an iodine-deficient body.

(4) Iodine is effective in treating fibrocystic breast disease. Iodine supplementation results in 70% improvement for fibrocystic breast disease.

(5) Iodine is beneficial for fibrocystic breast disease and prostate disease. Iodine's high dietary consumption in the Japanese likely explains their low incidence of breast and prostate disease.

(6) Iodine exerts anti-tumor effects against breast, thyroid, and prostate cancer.

(7) The increased prevalence of iodine deficiency in recent decades is likely the cause of an increase in breast cancer in the USA. In contrast, the high iodine consumption in Japanese women is likely responsible

for them having an exceptionally low incidence of breast cancer.

(8) A significant increase in iodine deficiency has occurred in the USA since the 1970s. The cause is likely the removal of iodine from bread and its substitution with bromine which further exacerbates iodine deficiency by competing with iodine receptors.

(9) Iodine deficiency explains the increasing incidence of breast cancer in young women in the USA. The high consumption of iodine by specific Asian populations, such as Japanese, correlates with a low incidence of breast and prostate diseases in those countries.

(10) The recommended dietary intake of iodine in the USA is 100 times too low. People in Japan consume 13.8-200 mg of iodine daily. This amount is 100-1,300 times the USA RDA of only 0.15 mg.

(11) Americans are consuming half as much iodine today compared to 30 years ago. One in seven American women develop breast cancer today compared to one in twenty women 30 years ago, an increase of 300%. The incidence of fibrocystic breast disease was 3% in the 1920s versus 90% today.

(12) The anticancer function of iodine may be one of its most important benefits. Other benefits are suppression of autoimmunity, strengthening the immune

system, and protecting against abnormal bacterial growth in the stomach.

(13) Iodine produces a greater sense of well-being, increased energy, clarity of thought, improved skin complexion, and more regular bowel movements. It also increases longevity.

(14) Cancer patients are very iodine deficient.

(15) Iodine deficiency risk is present in over 50% of pregnant women in New York City. This significantly increases the risk of autism and hearing loss in their children.

(16) Iodine deficient children have 6.9-10.2 points lower IQs. Severely iodine deficient children have 12.45 points lower IQs. Iodine deficiency in pregnant mothers can lower the IQs of the children by more than 30 points. Sufficient iodine can increase mental performance in children.

(17) Iodine deficiency is likely a cause of arrhythmias and congestive heart failure.

(18) Selenium supplementation is important when taking iodine because selenium deficiency is common, and selenium is necessary for normal thyroid and immune function.

(19) Magnesium is an important mineral for the immune system but magnesium deficiency is common worldwide.

(20) Calcium is an important mineral for the immune system but calcium deficiency is common worldwide.

Iodine is commercially available as Lugol's iodine solution in liquid or tablet form.

Dr. David Brownstein recommends that adults take 50 mg of iodine per day. This requires eight drops of Lugol's 5% iodine solution or twenty drops of Lugol's 2% iodine solution. Children should take a proportionate lesser amount based on weight. Lugol's 5% iodine solution contains ~6.25 mg of iodine per drop.

[Brownstein, D. (2009). *Iodine: Why You Need It, Why You Can't Live Without It* (4th Edition). West Bloomfield, Michigan: Medical Alternatives Press.]

A one-ounce bottle of Lugol's 5% iodine solution contains 600 drops which is enough for an adult for 2.5 months when taking eight drops daily, i.e., 50 mg daily. Lugol's iodine solution should be mixed with juice to avoid the metallic taste.

Lugol's iodine solution is available in some health food stores, on Amazon, and from other online providers such as Loudwolf Industrial and Scientific Company.

[Loudwolf. (2022). *Loudwolf Industrial and Scientific Company.* Loudwolf: Dublin, California. Retrieved 3 July 2022 https://www.loudwolf.com/]

Lugol's iodine solution is also available from J. Crow's Marketplace.

[J. Crow Co. (2022). *J. Crow's Marketplace.* J. Crow Co: New Ipswich, New Hampshire. Retrieved 3 July 2022 https://www.jcrowsmarketplace.com/]

Lugol's iodine is available in tablet form as Iodoral® by Optimox® on their website and on Amazon.

[Optimox. (2022). *Optimox.* Optimox: South Salt Lake, Utah. Retrieved 3 July 2022 https://www.optimox.com]

Part V: Diagnosis and Treatment of Warts

Chapter 27
Genital Warts

Genital warts refers to anogenital warts, condyloma acuminata, vaginal warts, penile warts, verruca acuminata, or venereal warts. Genital warts vary in appearance depending on location and stage of development. They can be tiny, light-colored dots initially. A full-blown genital wart is usually fleshy and raised significantly above the normal skin with a cauliflower appearance. Warts may bleed easily, be friable, and itch.

Warts can occur in singles, clumps, and multiple locations, including the genital area on or inside, the penis, vagina, anus, and the oral cavity. Genital warts occur in a small percentage of HPV infections. To be examined for genital warts, men should see a urologist, and women should see an Ob-Gyn doctor.

HPV types 6 and 11 are most commonly associated with anogenital warts.

Dr. Luisa Barzon and six medical colleagues at the Department of Histology of the University of Padova in Padova Italy published an article in the August 2010 issue of the *Journal of Medical Virology* concerning the prevalence of different HPV types. They examined 3,410 females and 1,033 males undergoing voluntary screening for HPV. Dr. Barzon said: "Anogenital warts were associated with HPV 6 and HPV 11 infection, and, less frequently, with other types, like HPV 54, HPV 62, and HPV 66."

[Barzon, L., et al. (2010). Distribution of human papillomavirus types in the anogenital tract of females and males. *J Med Virol. 2010 Aug; 82 (8): 1424-30.* https://pubmed.ncbi.nlm.nih.gov/20572068/]

Once infected by HPV, some women may develop genital warts, cervical or vaginal dysplasia, or both, depending to some extent on the HPV type. Other women may become HPV carriers with no signs or symptoms or eventually become immune to certain HPV types.

When men are infected by HPV, they may develop genital warts, become carriers, or may eventually become immune to certain HPV types.

Ninety percent of people infected with HPV do

not develop warts, and only 10% will transmit the virus.

Dr. Stephen W. Leslie at the Creighton University Medical Center in Omaha Nebraska, and two medical colleagues, published an article in the February 2022 issue of the *StatPearls* journal. They concluded that 90% of those contracting HPV will not develop genital warts. Only 10% who are infected by HPV will transmit the virus. Dr. Leslie noted that HPV types 6 and 11 are the most common types that cause genital warts.

[Leslie, S.W., et al. (2022). Genital Warts. Treasure Island, Florida: *StatPearls Publishing. February 14, 2022.* https://www.ncbi.nlm.nih.gov/books/NBK441884/]

HPV may be contagious even when warts and dysplasia are not detectable.

It is worthwhile to have an HPV test performed in all cases of suspected HPV.

HPV-negative tests do not rule out an HPV infection because (1) less than 10% of the known 228 HPV types are usually tested, and (2) the tests can yield false-negative results even for the few types tested. Therefore, treatment may be considered if HPV is suspected in the presence of HPV symptoms in the patient or the patient's partner.

Chapter 28
Plantar Warts, Palmar Warts, Flat Warts, and Common Warts

W arts are a widespread disease in all age
groups.

The prevalence of common and plantar warts in students was 22%.

Dr. M. Kilkenny at the University of Melbourne Department of Medicine in Victoria Australia, and two medical colleagues, published an article in the May 1998 issue of the *British Journal of Dermatology* in which the prevalence of common and plantar warts was evaluated. Among 2,491 students throughout Victoria Australia Dr. Kilkenny found that the overall prevalence of warts was 22%, varying from 12% in 4-6 year olds to 24% in 16-18 year olds. Common warts were the most frequent at 16% compared with plantar warts at 6% and plane, or flat, warts at only 2%. Dr. Kilkenny said:

Almost 40% of those found to have warts on examination had indicated on the survey questionnaire that they did not have any of these lesions. Of those who knew that they had warts, only 38% had used any treatment for them.

[Kilkenny, M., et al. (1998). The prevalence of common skin conditions in Australian school students: Common, plane and plantar viral warts. *Br J Dermatol. 1998 May; 138 (5): 840-5*. https://pubmed.ncbi.nlm.nih.gov/9666831/]

The prevalence of antibodies for patients with warts was 23.4% for HPV 1 and 41.5% for HPV 2.

Dr. K. Steele at the Department of General Practice of Queen's University in Belfast Ireland, and seven medical colleagues, published an article in the December 1988 issue of the *Epidemiology of Infections* journal. They studied the prevalence of antibodies in patients desiring treatment for warts. Dr. Steele found that among 376 patients screened for HPV types 1 and 2 antibodies, 23.4% of patients were positive for HPV type 1, and 41.5% were positive for HPV type 2. Dr. Steele said:

HPV 1 antibody was significantly more likely to be associated with plantar warts. HPV 2 antibody was present in 34.1% of patients with plantar warts and 45.6% of patients with warts at other sites. Evidence of multiple infection by HPV types 1 and 2 was demonstrated by the finding of HPV 1 and 2 antibodies in 4.3%.

[Steele, K., et al. (1988). A study of HPV 1, 2, and 4 antibody prevalence in patients presenting for treatment with cutaneous warts to general practitioners in N. Ireland. *Epidemiol Infect. 1988 Dec; 101 (3): 537-46.* https://pubmed.ncbi.nlm.nih.gov/2850937/]

The prevalence of antibodies to these HPV types indicates that the patients are developing immunity naturally.

HPV-negative tests do not rule out an HPV infection because (1) less than 10% of the known 228 HPV types are usually tested, and (2) the tests can yield false-negative results even for the few types tested. Therefore, treatment may be considered if HPV is suspected in the presence of HPV symptoms in the patient or the patient's partner.

Chapter 29
Medical and Surgical Treatments for Warts

A ldara cream 5%, also known as imiquimod, is a commonly used medical therapy for warts. Other medical treatments include podofilox (podophyllotoxin), sinecatechins, trichloracetic acid, and salicylic acid. Cryotherapy is used successfully for common warts but not for plantar warts.

Aldara 5% cream had 50% success eradicating genital warts in 4 months, but 13% had a recurrence of warts.

Dr. Libby Edwards and seven medical colleagues at the Department of Internal Medicine of Carolinas Medical Center in Charlotte North Carolina published an article in the January 1998 issue of the *Archives in Dermatology* journal on the success of Aldara cream for warts. Dr. Edwards reported that 311 patients with anogenital warts were in the study. 50% of the patients who received 5% imiquimod cream and 21% of those who received 1% imiquimod cream experienced eradication of all treated warts in 4 months. 13% of patients who received 5% imiquimod experienced a recurrence of at least one wart. Dr. Edwards said: "Five percent imiquimod cream is an effective and safe self-administered therapy for external anogenital warts when applied 3 times a week overnight for up to 16 weeks."

[Edwards, L., et al. (1998.) Self-administered topical 5% imiquimod cream for external anogenital warts. HPV Study Group. Human Papillomavirus. *Arch Dermatol. 1998 Jan; 134 (1): 25-30.* https://pubmed.ncbi.nlm. nih.gov/9449906/]

Podophyllotoxin was more effective in eradicating genital warts than imiquimod 5% cream but had more side effects.

Dr. J.M. Jung and six medical colleagues at the Department of Dermatology of the University of Ulsan College of Medicine in Seoul South Korea published an article in the July 2020 issue of the *British Journal of Dermatology*. They evaluated topical treatments of genital warts in 6,371 patients. Dr. Jung concluded:

Among conventional agents, podophyllotoxin was significantly more efficacious than imiquimod 5%

cream for lesion clearance; however, it was associated with a higher overall adverse event rate. Sinecatechins 15% ointment was significantly less efficacious than imiquimod 5% cream. None of the treatments were significantly different from each other with respect to recurrence, patients with severe adverse events, or patients who withdrew because of treatment-related adverse events. Conventional modalities were efficacious and well-tolerated, although each of them had their advantages and disadvantages.

[Jung, J.M., et al. (2020). Topically applied treatments for external genital warts in non-immunocompromised patients: a systematic review and network meta-analysis. *Br J Dermatol. 2020 Jul; 183 (1): 24-36.* https://pubmed.ncbi.nlm.nih.gov/31675442/]

Cryotherapy and salicylic acid are effective for common warts but have low success for plantar warts.

Dr. Sara Garcia-Oreja and five medical colleagues at the University Podiatric Clinic of the Complutense University of Madrid in Madrid Spain published an article in the January 2021 issue of the journal of *Dermatologic Therapy* about treatments for plantar warts. Dr. Garcia-Oreja said:

The average cure rates of the most frequent treatments were: cryotherapy (45.61%), salicylic acid (13.6%), cantharidin-podophyllin-salicylic acid formulation (97.82%), laser (79.36%), topical antivirals (72.45%), intralesional bleomycin (83.37%), and intralesional immunotherapy (68.14%). First-choice treatments for common warts, such as cryotherapy and salicylic acid, have low-cure rates for plantar warts.

[Garcia-Oreja, S., et al. (2021). Topical treatment for plantar warts: A systematic review. *Dermatol Ther. 2021 Jan; 34 (1): e14621.* https://pubmed.ncbi.nlm.nih.gov/ 33263934/]

Traditional treatments for warts each had their benefits and disadvantages.

According to testimonial evidence, Betamannan™ has a 95% success for warts when treated for three months, with no side effects.

Chapter 30
Comparison of Wart Treatments

A ny topical wart treatment will be more effective if one of the warts is gently filed daily with a mild fingernail file before application of treatment. However, do not file a facial wart.

The objective is not to eliminate the wart with the file but to help expose the HPV to the immune cells by disrupting HPV-containing skin cells. No filing should be done on facial warts. Only one wart needs to be treated with filing since all the other warts will disappear once immunity develops.

(1) Imiquimod, also known as Aldara cream, has a 21-50% success but had a 13% recurrence rate within three months. Therefore the real success for Aldara cream was 37% using the 5% concentration of

Aldara cream. Side effects include skin redness, fatigue, body aches, blisters, and rash.

(2) According to testimonial evidence, Beta-mannan™ has a 95% success when treating warts for three months, with no side effects.

The natural history of the disease would predict a 70% cure rate in 2 years, whereas Beta-mannan™ has a 95% cure rate in 3 months.

Immunity to HPV is acquired frequently.

Immunity to HPV must specify a particular HPV type - one of the 228 currently identified. If a person tests positive for a particular type or types, but later tests negative for them, then that person has achieved immunity for those particular types, assuming the test result is not a false-negative result.

HPV-negative tests do not rule out an HPV infection because (1) less than 10% of the known 228 HPV types are usually tested, and (2) the tests can yield false-negative results even for the few types tested. Therefore, treatment may be considered if HPV is suspected in the presence of HPV symptoms in the patient or the patient's partner.

Chapter 31
Pearly Penile Papules

Pearly penile papules are occasionally misdiagnosed as genital warts but are merely a normal anatomical variant in men. They appear as small, dome-shaped to filiform skin-colored papules typically located on the sulcus or corona of the glans penis. Lesions are generally arranged circumferentially in one or several rows.

Pearly penile papules have no malignant potential. They are not contracted or spread through sexual activity; however, the mechanisms underlying their development remain unknown. Pearly penile papules are commonly noted in males in their second or third decades of life, with a gradual decrease in frequency with aging.

Pearly penile papules were found in 48% of men.

Dr. C. Sonnet and Dr. W.G. Dockerty at the Department of Genitourinary Medicine of Addenbrooke's Hospital in Cambridge England published an article in the November 1999 issue of the *International Journal of STD and AIDS*. A study of 200 men found a prevalence of pearly penile papules in 48%. 73% of the men had only a few less than 1 mm lesions, but 8% had lesions greater than 1 mm in size extending around the corona. Several of the men underwent laser ablation surgery with good cosmetic results. Dr. Sonnet said: "Over one-third of men with papules had previously been concerned or worried by their presence, and approximately one-quarter had experienced embarrassment."

[Sonnex, C., et al. (1999). Pearly penile papules: a common cause of concern. *Int J STD AIDS. 1999 Nov; 10 (11):* 726-7. https://pubmed.ncbi.nlm.nih.gov/ 10563558/]

HPV was not found in pearly penile papules.

Dr. A. Ferenczy and two medical colleagues at the Department of Pathology of Sir Mortimer B. Davis Jewish General Hospital in Montreal Quebec Canada published an article in the July 1991 issue of the *Obstetrics and Gynecology* journal. They examined biopsy specimens for HPV from 13 men with pearly penile papules. Dr. Ferenczy said: "None of the pearly penile papules contained HPV DNA sequences."

[Ferenczy, A., et al. (1991). Pearly penile papules: absence of human papillomavirus DNA by the polymerase chain reaction. *Obstet Gynecol. 1991 Jul; 78 (1): 118-22.* https://pubmed.ncbi.nlm.nih.gov/2047052/]

Cryotherapy and laser therapy are two reliable cosmetic treatments for pearly penile papules.

Dr. Adam S. Aldahan and two medical colleagues at the University of Miami Miller School of Medicine in Miami Florida published an article in the May 2018 issue of the *American Journal of Men's Health* describing the diagnosis and management of pearly penile papules. Dr. Aldahan noted that despite their benign nature, pearly penile papules are known to cause significant emotional distress because they resemble genital warts. Dr. Aldahan said: "For patients who still desire treatment after counseling, cryotherapy and laser therapy represent two reliable treatment options with low rates of recurrence."

[Aldahan, A.S., et al. (2016). Diagnosis and management of pearly penile papules. *Am J Mens Health. 2018 May; 12 (3): 624-627.* https://www.ncbi.nlm.nih.gov/pmc/articles/PMC5987947/]

Therefore, although there is no risk of cancer or HPV in cases of pearly penile papules, some men may wish to have them removed for cosmetic reasons.

Chapter 32
Molluscum Contagiosum

Molluscum contagiosum, unrelated to HPV, is occasionally misdiagnosed as warts. Molluscum is a common viral infection of the skin, more common in children. It is caused by a DNA virus of the poxvirus group. The lesions are discrete, pearly, skin-colored, dome-shaped papules varying in size from 1 to 5 mm. Typically they have central umbilication from which a plug of cheesy material can be expressed; however, expression of these plugs should be avoided as it will result in deep scarring. These papules may occur anywhere, but the face, eyelids, neck, underarms, and thighs are the most common sites of infection. Lesions may also occur in clusters on the genitalia or in the groin of adolescents. Mucosal lesions are rare.

A variety of factors should determine the course of treatment for molluscum contagiosum.

Dr. Alexander K.C. Leung at the Alberta Children's Hospital of the University of Calgary in Calgary Alberta Canada, and two medical colleagues, published an article in the 2017 issue of *Recent Patents on Inflammation and Allergy Drug Discoveries* journal about molluscum contagiosum. Dr. Leung said:

> The choice of treatment method should depend on the physician's comfort level with the various treatment options, the patient's age, the number and severity of lesions, location of lesions, and the preference of the child and parents.

[Leung, A.K.C., et al. (2017). Molluscum contagiosum: an update. *Recent Pat Inflamm Allergy Drug Discov. 2017; 11 (1): 22-31.* https://pubmed.ncbi.nlm.nih.gov/28521677/]

Molluscum contagiosum is a self-limited disease, but lesions can persist for months to years, spread to distant sites, and be transmitted to others.

Molluscum contagiosum resolved in 46% in 16 weeks with imiquimod treatment.

Dr. Elizabeth Liota and four medical colleagues at the Department of Dermatology of the National Naval

Medical Center in Bethesda Maryland published an article in the April 2000 issue of the *Journal of Cutaneous Medicine and Surgery* to study the use of imiquimod for molluscum contagiosum. Dr. Liota found that 6 of 13 children, or 46%, had resolution of their molluscum lesions with 16 weeks of imiquimod therapy.

[Liota, E., et al. (2000). Imiquimod therapy for molluscum contagiosum. *J Cutan Med Surg. 2000 Apr; 4 (2): 76-82.* https://pubmed.ncbi.nlm.nih.gov/11179929/]

Molluscum contagiosum has responded to some of the same treatments as genital warts.

Part VI: Men and HPV

Chapter 33
Men and HPV-related Diseases

HPV has numerous types. Some types, such as HPV 6 or 11, are more frequently associated with common, plantar, flat, and anogenital warts. Other types such as HPV 16 or 18 are more frequently associated with cervical dysplasia.

In men, genital warts are the most frequent clinical manifestation of HPV and are readily visible to the naked eye. Warts can cause considerable discomfort, irritation, and bleeding. Anogenital warts generally occur on the penis or anal region. HPV is only rarely associated with any type of cancerous lesion in men.

Anal and oral lesions, as well as penile carcinoma, may be caused by HPV.

Dr. Laura Sichero at the Center for Translational Research in Oncology of the Faculdade de Medicina da

Universidade de São Paulo in São Paulo Brazil, and two medical colleagues, published an article in the 2019 issue of the *Acta Cytologica* journal about HPV in men. Dr. Sichero said:

> It is currently recognized that in addition to the major impact of human papillomavirus infection in females, HPV causes considerable disease in men at the genitals, anal canal, and oropharynx. Specifically, genital HPV infections may progress to genital warts and penile carcinoma.

[Sichero, L., et al. (2019). Human papillomavirus and genital disease in men: what we have learned from the HIM study. *Acta Cytol. 2019; 63 (2): 109-117.* https://pubmed.ncbi.nlm.nih.gov/30799416/]

HPV was found in 28.2% of men attending an STD clinic versus approximately 13% in the general population.

Dr. Susie B. Baldwin and eight medical colleagues at the Department of Obstetrics and Gynecology of the University of Arizona in Tucson Arizona published an article in the April 2003 issue of the *Journal of Infectious Diseases* about HPV in men attending an STD clinic. The prevalence of HPV was 28.2%. Multiple HPV types were found in 6.1% of participants, and unknown types in 5.9%.

[Baldwin, S.B., et al. (2003). Human papillomavirus infection in men attending a sexually transmitted disease clinic. *J Infect Dis. 2003 Apr 1; 187 (7): 1064-70.* https://pubmed.ncbi.nlm.nih.gov/12660920/]

Many methods have been found helpful for HPV detection in men, but none are approved by the FDA.

Dr. A. Vives at the Unidad de Andrología of the Universitat Autònoma de Barcelona in Barcelona Spain, and two medical colleagues, published an article in the March 2020 issue of the *Actas Urológicas Españolas* journal. It was an exhaustive review of the literature on HPV testing in men. Dr. Vives said:

No HPV test for men has been approved by the FDA, nor has any test been approved for detection of the virus in areas other than the cervix. Many methods for HPV detection have shown their usefulness in some of the pathologies associated with male HPV but, despite this, none of them has been approved for men.

[Vives, A., et al. (2020). The role of human papillomavirus test in men: First exhaustive review of literature. *Actas Urol Esp (Engl Ed). 2020 Mar; 44 (2): 86-93.* https://pubmed.ncbi.nlm.nih.gov/31874781/]

The diagnosis of genital warts in men usually requires a visible characteristic wart, a biopsy of a non-characteristic wart, or an HPV test of a biopsy specimen, penile urethral swab, or skin swab. A urologist is the proper specialist to examine men for genital warts.

HPV-negative tests do not rule out an HPV infection because (1) less than 10% of the known 228 HPV types are usually tested, and (2) the tests can yield false-negative results even for the few types tested. Therefore, treatment may be considered if HPV is suspected in the presence of HPV symptoms in the patient or the patient's partner.

Chapter 34
Partner Infections and HPV-related Considerations

Many women ask if their partners can keep reinfecting them after the woman is cured of cervical dysplasia or genital warts and if their partners should be treated.

If a woman develops immunity, she cannot catch the same HPV type from her partner and is no longer contagious for that HPV type. She is cured of that HPV type. However, if she does not develop immunity, she will still have HPV. Either way, her partner's status will not affect her unless he transmits a new HPV type to her.

Sex with a man who has the same HPV type as the woman will not cause reinfection of the woman after she has developed immunity to that type.

A woman cannot get reinfected by having sex with a

partner with the same HPV type to which she has already developed immunity.

HPV viruses should be viewed like common cold viruses concerning immunity. Once a woman gets over a common cold, she has developed immunity to one of over 300 common cold viruses and will not be infected by that same cold virus again.

If a man's partner has cervical dysplasia or genital warts, then there is a good chance that the man is a carrier or is immune to the same HPV type infecting his partner. Nevertheless, it is impossible to prove that he has HPV unless he has visible genital warts or a positive HPV test on a penile urethral swab performed by a urologist. However, even if the warts are not present and the HPV test is negative, it does not prove that he does not have HPV.

HPV-negative tests do not rule out an HPV infection because (1) less than 10% of the known 228 HPV types are usually tested, and (2) the tests can yield false-negative results even for the few types tested. Therefore, treatment may be considered if HPV is suspected in the presence of HPV symptoms in the patient or the patient's partner.

Chapter 35
Penile Cancer

HPV has been associated with cancer of the penis. For this reason, known cases of HPV infection in men are probably worth treating, although cancer of the penis is relatively rare.

HPV has been found in up to 92% of penile cancers.

Dr. M.R. Cupp and four medical colleagues at the Department of Urology of the Mayo Clinic in Rochester Minnesota published an article in the September 1995 issue of the *Journal of Urology* concerning the detection of HPV in cancer of the penis. Dr. Cupp detected HPV in 92% of carcinoma in situ and 92% of penile intraepithelial neoplasia, which are non-invasive. HPV 16 was the most common. Dr. Cupp said:

Overall, the detection rates for human papillomavirus were 55% for invasive squamous cell carcinoma, 92% for carcinoma in situ, and 92% for penile intraepithelial neoplasia. Moreover, the prevalence is greater in noninvasive lesions (carcinoma in situ and penile intraepithelial neoplasia) than in invasive carcinoma.

[Cupp, M.R., et al. (1995). The detection of human papillomavirus deoxyribonucleic acid in intraepithelial, in situ, verrucous, and invasive carcinoma of the penis. *J Urol. 1995 Sep; 154 (3): 1024-9.* https://pubmed.ncbi. nlm.nih.gov/7637047/]

The higher prevalence of HPV found in noninvasive lesions is likely due to a decreased immune response before invasion. When cancer becomes invasive, more HPV virus is exposed to an increased inflammatory response. This increased inflammatory response is more likely to permit the development of HPV immunity. However, once cancer has become invasive, it will usually progress even after an immune response eliminates HPV.

This study has demonstrated an association of HPV with penile cancer. It is worthwhile to have an HPV test performed in all cases of suspected HPV.

HPV-negative tests do not rule out an HPV infection because (1) less than 10% of the known 228 HPV types

are usually tested, and (2) the tests can yield false-negative results even for the few types tested. Therefore, treatment may be considered if HPV is suspected in the presence of HPV symptoms in the patient or the patient's partner.

Chapter 36
Prostate Disease and Prostate Cancer

The exact role of HPV in the development of benign and malignant lesions of the prostate is unclear.

BPH is an acronym for "**B**enign **P**rostatic **H**yperplasia" or "**B**enign **P**rostatic **H**ypertrophy" and refers to prostate gland enlargement.

Several studies have demonstrated an association of HPV with prostate disease, including prostate cancer. For this reason, treating men who are possible carriers of HPV takes on greater significance.

HPV infection significantly increases the risk of prostate cancer.

Dr. Binbin Yin at the Department of Laboratory Medicine of Zhejiang University School of Medicine in Zhejiang China, and ten medical colleagues, published an article in the August 2017 issue of the *Oncology Letters* journal on the occurrence of HPV and prostate cancer. Dr. Yin said: "The overall results provided evidence that HPV infection significantly increased the risk of prostate cancer."

[Yin, B., et al. (2017). Association between human papillomavirus and prostate cancer: A meta-analysis. *Oncol Lett. 2017 Aug; 14 (2): 1855–1865.* https://www. ncbi.nlm.nih.gov/pmc/articles/PMC5529902/]

HPV was found in 16-53% of prostate cancers.

Dr. Hiroyoshi Suzuki and four medical colleagues at the Department of Urology of the School of Medicine of Chiba University in Chiba-shi Japan published an article in the May 1996 issue of the *Prostate* journal. Dr. Suzuki found that HPV was detected in 16% of prostate cancer specimens.

[Suzuki, H., et al. (1996). Detection of human papillomavirus DNA and p53 gene mutations in human prostate cancer. *Prostate. 1996 May; 28 (5): 318-24.* https://pubmed.ncbi.nlm.nih.gov/8610059/]

Dr. Jurgen Serth, Dr. Frank Panitz, and three medical colleagues at the Department of Urology of Hannover Medical School in Hanover Germany published an article in the February 1999 issue of the journal of *Cancer Research*. Dr. Serth found that 21% of prostate cancers had HPV 16.

[Serth, J., et al. (1999). Increased levels of human papillomavirus type 16 DNA in a subset of prostate cancers. *Cancer Res 1999 Feb 15; 59 (4): 823-5.* https://pubmed.ncbi.nlm.nih.gov/10029070/]

Dr. Caroline Moyret-Lalle at the Institut de Genetique Moleculaire de Montpellier in Montpellier France, and eight medical colleagues, published an article in the April 1995 issue of the *International Journal of Cancer*. Dr. Moyret-Lalle said regarding prostate cancer: "53% of carcinomas were HPV 16."

[Moyret-Lalle, C., et al. (1995). Ras, p53 and HPV status in benign and malignant prostate tumors. *Int J Cancer. 1995 Apr 21; 64 (2): 124-9.* https://pubmed.ncbi.nlm.nih.gov/7542226/]

HPV was found in 93% of the cases of benign prostatic hyperplasia and in all four prostate cancers examined.

Dr. P.J. McNicol and Dr. J.G. Dodd at the Cadham Provincial Laboratory in Winnipeg in Manitoba Canada published an article in the March 1990 issue of the *Journal of Clinical Microbiology* describing HPV in prostate tissue. HPV 16 was found in 14 of 15, or 93%, of benign prostatic hyperplasias and all four, or 100%, of prostate cancers tested. In contrast, HPV 18 was identified in only three benign hyperplasias, which also contained HPV 16. Four of five normal prostates demonstrated no HPV infection. The presence of these HPV types in prostate tissues suggests an HPV reservoir for transmission.

[McNicol, P.J., et al. (1990). Detection of human papillomavirus DNA in prostate gland tissue by using the polymerase chain reaction amplification assay. *J Clin Microbiol. 1990 Mar; 28 (3): 409-12.* https://pubmed.ncbi.nlm.nih.gov/1691205/]

These studies have demonstrated an association of HPV with prostate cancer and benign prostatic hyperplasia. It is worthwhile to have an HPV test performed in all cases of suspected HPV.

HPV-negative tests do not rule out an HPV infection because (1) less than 10% of the known 228 HPV types are usually tested, and (2) the tests can yield false-negative results even for the few types tested. Therefore, treatment may be considered if HPV is suspected in the presence of HPV symptoms in the patient or the patient's partner.

Part VII: HPV-associated Conditions

Chapter 37
Infertility

HPV infections and cervical dysplasia may decrease fertility simply by preventing penetration of the sperm into the cervical canal. The cervical opening is small. HPV may cause chronic cervical inflammation that blocks the sperm's entry into the cervix. Sperm may not be able to penetrate the inflamed cervical opening effectively if the opening is full of white blood cells fighting HPV infection.

HPV infection was detected in 10-35.7% of infertile men's semen and was associated with anti-sperm antibodies and a decrease in sperm motility.

Dr. Carlo Foresta and three medical colleagues at the Department of Medicine and Centre for Human Reproduction Pathology of the University of Padova in Padova Italy published an article in the March 2015 issue of *Andrology* about HPV sperm infection and infertility. Dr. Foresta said:

> The prevalence of HPV sperm infection ranges between 2 and 31% in men from the general population and between 10 and 35.7% in men affected by unexplained infertility. The presence of HPV in semen is associated with an impairment of sperm motility and the presence of anti-sperm antibodies.

[Foresta, C., et al. (2015). HPV-DNA sperm infection and infertility: from a systematic literature review to a possible clinical management proposal. *Andrology. 2015 Mar; 3 (2): 163-73.* https://pubmed.ncbi.nlm.nih.gov/25270519/]

HPV infection is strongly associated with female infertility.

Dr. Shuang Yuan at the Department of Gynecology and Obstetrics of Sichuan University in Chengdu Sichuan Province China, and three medical colleagues, published an article in the February 2020 issue of the journal of *Reproductive Biomedicine Online*. Dr. Yuan reported the HPV effects on female infertility. He found six studies with a total of 11,869 participants showed a strong HPV association with female infertility and concluded that HPV infection is a definite risk factor.

[Yuan, S., et al. (2019). Human papillomavirus infection and female infertility: a systematic review and meta-analysis. *Reprod Biomed Online. 2020 Feb; 40 (2): 229-237.* https://pubmed.ncbi.nlm.nih.gov/31987733/]

These studies have demonstrated an association of HPV with infertility in both men and women. It is worthwhile to have an HPV test performed in all cases of suspected HPV.

HPV-negative tests do not rule out an HPV infection because (1) less than 10% of the known 228 HPV types are usually tested, and (2) the tests can yield false-negative results even for the few types tested. Therefore, treatment may be considered if HPV is suspected in the presence of HPV symptoms in the patient or the patient's partner.

Chapter 38
Miscarriages

HPV has been linked to spontaneous abortions or miscarriages. So the treatment of HPV is likely a way to prevent some spontaneous abortions or miscarriages.

HPV infection is very prevalent in miscarriages, particularly in early pregnancy. It was found in 60% of first trimester miscarriages - a significantly higher percentage than approximately 13% found in the general population. Furthermore, 100% of third trimester healthy placentas had no HPV infection.

Dr. Hermonat and three medical colleagues at the Department of Obstetrics and Gynecology of the University of Arkansas for Medical Sciences in Little Rock Arkansas published an article in the February 1998 issue of the *Human Pathology* journal. It examined the incidence of HPV in spontaneous abortions. Dr. Hermonat found that HPV infection was three times more prevalent in spontaneous abortion specimens compared with elective specimens. Furthermore, all 4 of 4 third trimester placentas examined had no HPV infection. This suggests that HPV-infected placentas may have altered characteristics, leading to a miscarriage in early pregnancy.

[Hermonat, P.L., et al. (1998). Trophoblasts are the preferential target for human papillomavirus infection in spontaneously aborted. *Hum Pathol. 1998 Feb; 29 (2):* 170-4. https://pubmed.ncbi.nlm.nih.gov/9490277/]

Dr. Lukasz Bober at the Medical University of Lodz in Lodz Poland, and three medical colleagues, published an article in the 2019 issue of the journal of *Ginekologia Polska*. It concerned the effect of HPV on early pregnancy. These doctors concluded that HPV in early pregnancy might cause miscarriage in their study of 143 pregnant women. HPV infection was more frequent in patients with an abnormal course in the first trimester of pregnancy. Dr. Bober said: "The obtained results may confirm the presence of adverse effects of HPV infection on early pregnancy."

[Bober, L., et al. (2019). Influence of human papillomavirus (HPV) infection on early pregnancy. *Ginekol*

Pol. 2019; 90 (2): 72-75. https://pubmed.ncbi.nlm.nih.gov/30860272/]

Dr. P.L. Hermonat and six medical colleagues at the University of Arkansas Medical Sciences in Little Rock Arkansas published an article in the 1997 issue of the *Virus Genes* journal. Dr. Hermonat found HPV to be much more prevalent in spontaneous abortions. 60% of spontaneous abortion placentas were infected with HPV. These results suggest the possibility that HPV may be the cause of some spontaneous abortions.

[Hermonat, P.L., et al. (1997). Human papillomavirus is more prevalent in first trimester spontaneously aborted specimens. *Virus Genes. 1997; 14 (1): 13-7.* https://pubmed.ncbi.nlm.nih.gov/9208451/]

These studies have demonstrated an association of HPV with miscarriages. It is worthwhile to have an HPV test performed in all cases of suspected HPV.

HPV-negative tests do not rule out an HPV infection because (1) less than 10% of the known 228 HPV types are usually tested, and (2) the tests can yield false-negative results even for the few types tested. Therefore, treatment may be considered if HPV is suspected in the presence of HPV symptoms in the patient or the patient's partner.

Chapter 39
Oral Lesions

C ircumvallate papillae are commonly mistaken for oral HPV warts. These papillae are arranged in an inverted V at the back of the tongue. These papillae are evenly distributed on the back of the tongue in an organized fashion and are part of the normal anatomy. These are not to be confused with oral warts.

HPV oral infection was present in 12.5% of oral cancer patients, 27.3% of lichen planus patients, and 29.6% of leukoplakia patients.

Dr. L. Sand and three medical colleagues at the Department of Oral and Maxillofacial Surgery of the Goteborg University in Goteborg Sweden published an article in the March 2000 issue of the *Anticancer Research* journal about HPV in oral lesions. Dr. Sand found that 12.5% of oral cancer biopsies were HPV-positive. 27.3% of lichen planus patients were HPV-positive. And 29.6% of patients with leukoplakia were HPV-positive. Notice that the prevalence of HPV infection was higher in the less advanced stages of the disease. This supports the theory that once cancer develops and causes more inflammation, it is more likely that the patient will develop immunity to the HPV and therefore test HPV-negative.

[Sand, L., et al. (2000). Human papillomaviruses in oral lesions. *Anticancer Res.* Mar-Apr 2000; 20 (2B): 1183-8. https://pubmed.ncbi.nlm.nih.gov/10810419/]

The average time of clearance of HPV oral infections was 46 days.

Dr. Andrew F. Brouwer at the Department of Epidemiology of the University of Michigan in Ann Arbor Michigan, and twelve medical colleagues, published an article in the January 2022 issue of the *British Medical Journal.* It compared oral and genital HPV infections. Dr. Brouwer reported that oral HPV infections were transient, with only 16% persisting to the next clinic visit. The average time for oral HPV infection to clear was 46 days. In contrast, genital HPV infections lasted longer, with 56% persisting to the next clinic visit. The average time for genital HPV infection to clear was 87 days. In conclusion, Dr. Brouwer noted that oral HPV was highly transient, and the incidence was associated with recent deep kissing and two or more sexual partners.

[Brouwer, A.F., et al. (2022). Incidence and clearance of oral and cervicogenital HPV infection: longitudinal analysis of the MHOC cohort study. *BMJ Open. 2022 Jan 3; 12 (1): e056502.* https://pubmed.ncbi.nlm.nih.gov/34980629/]

HPV oral lesions are rare, most of which are cleared within one year.

Dr. Aimee R. Kreimer at the National Cancer Institute of the National Institutes of Health in Bethesda Maryland, and ten medical colleagues, published an article in the July 2013 issue of the *Lancet* journal. The study consisted of 1,626 men with oral HPV infections. Dr. Kreimer said:

During the first 12 months of follow-up, 4.4% of men acquired an incident oral HPV infection. Median duration of infection was 6.9 months. Newly acquired oral oncogenic HPV infections in healthy men were rare, and most were cleared within 1 year.

[Kreimer, A.R., et al. (2013). Incidence and clearance of oral human papillomavirus infection in men: the HIM cohort study. *Lancet. 2013 Sep 7; 382 (9895): 877–*

887. https://www.ncbi.nlm.nih.gov/pmc/articles/ PMC3904652/]

Dr. Chaoting Zhang at the Key Laboratory of Carcinogenesis of Peking University Cancer Hospital in Beijing China, and thirteen medical colleagues, published an article in the August 2017 issue of the *Oncotarget* journal. Dr. Zhang reported on the natural history of oral HPV and said: "Most newly acquired infections were cleared within one year. Recent practice of oral sex increased the risk of incident infection. Newly acquired oral mucosal HPV infections are rare."

[Zhang, C., et al. (2017). Incidence and clearance of oral human papillomavirus infection: A population-based cohort study in rural China. *Oncotarget. 2017 Aug 29; 8 (35): 59831–59844.* https://www.ncbi.nlm.nih. gov/pmc/articles/PMC5601782/]

Oral HPV infections are rare even among women with HPV-positive Pap smears and also rare among the partners of these women.

Dr. T.K. Eggersmann at the Department of Obstetrics and Gynecology and Breast Center of the University of Munich in Munich Germany, and ten medical colleagues, published an article in the June 2019 issue of the *Archives of Gynecology and Obstetrics* journal. The article discussed oral HPV in women and included 144

HPV-positive women, 77 HPV-negative women, and 157 sexual partners. Dr. Eggersmann reported:

> The present study aims to determine the prevalence of oral HPV infection in cervical HPV-positive and negative women and their sexual partners. One woman with an HPV-positive cervical smear and one partner of a woman with an HPV-positive cervical smear showed an oral HPV infection. No oral HPV infections were detected in the HPV-negative control group. The overall incidence of oral HPV infection was 0.5%, and the incidence of oral HPV infection in women with a positive cervical smear was 0.7%. The data demonstrate that the overall risk of an oral HPV infection is low. HPV transmission to the oropharynx by auto-inoculation or oral-genital contact constitutes a rare and unlikely event.

[Eggersmann, T.K., et al. (2019). Prevalence of oral HPV infection in cervical HPV-positive women and their sexual partners. *Arch Gynecol Obstet. 2019 Jun; 299 (6): 1659-1665.* https://pubmed.ncbi.nlm.nih.gov/30953186/]

Oral HPV is rare in men and women, and it usually clears within a year. However, HPV may rarely cause oral cancers.

HPV-negative tests do not rule out an HPV infection because (1) less than 10% of the known 228 HPV types are usually tested, and (2) the tests can yield false-negative results even for the few types tested. Therefore, treatment may be considered if HPV is suspected in the presence of HPV symptoms in the patient or the patient's partner

Chapter 40
Anal Cancer

Infection with HPV is associated with anal cancer.

A Pap smear of anal cells is called anal cytology, whereas a Pap smear of cervical cells is called cervical cytology.

HPV was detected in 92% of anal cancers.

Dr. N. Ouhoummane and seven medical colleagues at the Institut National de Santé Publique du Québec in Montréal Quebec Canada published an article in the December 2013 issue of the *Cancer Epidemiology* journal about anal cancer and HPV. Dr. Ouhoummane said:

> Among the 606 patients with anal cancers, HPV was detected in 92% of cases. HPV 16 was the most frequent type detected in 90% of HPV-positive speci-

mens. Other types including 6, 11, 18, 33, 52, 53, 56, 58, 62, and 82 were also found. HPV infection, especially HPV 16, is strongly associated with squamous anal cancer.

[Ouhoummane, N., et al. (2013). Squamous anal cancer: patient characteristics and HPV type distribution. *Cancer Epidemiol.* 2013 Dec; 37 (6): 807-12. https://pubmed.ncbi.nlm.nih.gov/24139594/]

Abnormal anal cytology was found in 3.9% of young women. The risk was highest in women with abnormal Pap smears or those who engaged in anal intercourse.

Dr. Anna-Barbara Mosciki and nine medical colleagues at the Department of Pediatrics of the University of California in San Francisco California published an article in the February 1999 issue of the journal of *Cancer Epidemiological Biomarkers Preview.* They studied risk factors for abnormal anal smears in young women. Dr. Mosciki found that anal cancers are four times more common in women than men. There were 410 women with an average age of 22 years who were in the study for one year. 3.9% were found to have abnormal anal cytology smears. Factors significantly associated with abnormal anal cytology were a history of anal sex, abnormal Pap smears, and a current anal

HPV infection. Dr. Mosciki said: "Young women who had engaged in anal intercourse or had a history of cervical SILs were found to be at highest risk."

[Moscicki, A.B., et al. (1999). Risk factors for abnormal anal cytology in young heterosexual women. *Cancer Epidemiol Biomarkers Prev. 1999 Feb; 8 (2): 173-8.* https://pubmed.ncbi.nlm.nih.gov/10067816/]

Most untreated anal HPV infections cleared within three years.

Dr. Anna-Barbara Moscicki and nine medical colleagues at the Department of Pediatrics of the University of California in San Francisco California published an article in the March 2014 issue of the *Clinical Infectious Diseases* journal about the natural history of anal HPV in women. These doctors reported that 75 women with anal HPV were in the study. Dr. Moscicki said: "The majority of anal HPV infections cleared within 3 years. HPV-16 infections were slower to clear than other HR-HPV infections, consistent with its role in anal cancer."

[Moscicki, A.B., et al. (2014). Natural history of anal human papillomavirus infection in heterosexual women and risks associated with persistence. *Clin Infect Dis. 2014 Mar; 58 (6): 804-11.* https://pubmed.ncbi.nlm.nih.gov/24368624/]

Abnormal anal cytology was found in 5.5% of women with abnormal cervical cytology.

Dr. Perapong Inthasorn at the Department of Obstetrics and Gynaecology of Mahidol University in Bangkok Thailand, and five medical colleagues, published an article in the July 2021 issue of the *Asian Pacific Journal of Cancer Prevention*. Dr. Inthasorn reported on the prevalence of abnormal anal cytology and said:

> The aim of this study was to evaluate the prevalence of abnormal anal cytology in women presenting with abnormal cervical cytology. Anal cytology was performed on 145 women with abnormal cervical cytology. Prevalence of abnormal anal cytology was 5.5% in patients with abnormal cervical cytology. The prevalence might support anal cytology screening in this group of patients.

[Inthasorn, P., et al. (2021). Prevalence of abnormal anal cytology in women with abnormal cervical cytology. *Asian Pac J Cancer Prev. 2021 Jul 1; 22 (7): 2165-2169.* https://pubmed.ncbi.nlm.nih.gov/34319039/]

HPV-negative tests do not rule out an HPV infection because (1) less than 10% of the known 228 HPV types

are usually tested, and (2) the tests can yield false-negative results even for the few types tested. Therefore, treatment may be considered if HPV is suspected in the presence of HPV symptoms in the patient or the patient's partner.

Chapter 41
Urethritis

HPV has been detected in studies of chronic urinary tract infections also known as chronic urethritis. In these cases, HPV likely plays a significant role. HPV may create an environment encouraging the persistence of other bacterial infectious agents such as *Chlamydia trachomatis*, *Mycoplasma*, and *Ureaplasma*.

HPV was found in 31-48% of men with urethritis - a significantly higher percentage than approximately 13% found in the general population.

Dr. F. Chiarini and Dr. S. Pisani and eight medical colleagues at the School of Medicine of the University of Rome in Rome Italy published an article in the December 1998 issue of the *Minerva Urology and Nephrology* journal. It described the detection of HPV in men with chronic urethritis. Dr. Chiarini said: "Genital

HPV was detected in 31% of specimens positive for two or more agents."

[Chiarini, F., et al. (1998). Simultaneous detection of HPV and other sexually transmitted agents in chronic urethritis. *Minerva Urol Nefrol. 1998 Dec; 50 (4): 225-31.* https://pubmed.ncbi.nlm.nih.gov/9973807/]

Dr. Kazuyoshi Shigehara and eight medical colleagues at the Kanazawa University Graduate School of Medical Science in Ishikawa Japan published an article in the June 2010 issue of the *International Journal of Urology.* It concerned the incidence of HPV in men with urethritis. These doctors reported that of 142 men with urethritis, HPV was detected in 48%, and high-risk HPV was found in 32%. They concluded that the urinary tract is frequently infected by HPV in men with urethritis.

[Shigehara, K., et al. (2010). Prevalence of human papillomavirus infection in the urinary tract of men with urethritis. *Int J Urol. 2010 Jun; 17 (6): 563-8.* https://pubmed.ncbi.nlm.nih.gov/20345431/]

HPV 16 was found in the urinary tract of 75% of biopsies from women with persistent urethritis and cystitis.

Dr. A.M. Agliano at the Department of Experimental Medicine of Sapienza University in Rome Italy, and eight medical colleagues, published an article in the 1994 issue of the journal of *Urologia Internationalis*. The article reported the detection of HPV 16 in 75% of female urinary tracts with persistent urethritis and cystitis. Dr. Agliano said:

> We investigated the presence of human papillomavirus-related DNA sequences (HPV 6, 11, 16, and 18) in 33 biopsies from the urinary tracts of female patients with recurrent and persistent urethritis and cystitis. Sequences homologous to HPV 6, 11, and 18 genomes were not found, while HPV 16-related DNA sequences were identified in 25 of 33 lesions with histopathological diagnosis of metaplasia. The results suggest that the spread of HPV in the female urinary tract may not be uncommon and point to the need for further research on the possible pathogenic role in recurrent female disturbances.

[Agliano, A.M., et al. (1994). Detection of human papillomavirus type 16 DNA sequences in paraffin-embedded tissues from the female urinary tract. *Urol Int. 1994; 52 (4): 208-12.* https://pubmed.ncbi.nlm.nih.gov/8030168/]

These studies have demonstrated an association of HPV with urethritis in both men and women. It is worthwhile to have an HPV test performed in all cases of suspected HPV.

HPV-negative tests do not rule out an HPV infection because (1) less than 10% of the known 228 HPV types are usually tested, and (2) the tests can yield false-negative results even for the few types tested. Therefore, treatment may be considered if HPV is suspected in the presence of HPV symptoms in the patient or the patient's partner.

Chapter 42
Vaginosis

HPV is associated with vaginosis. This is commonly diagnosed as bacterial vaginosis, also called BV.

Bacterial vaginosis is believed to be caused by *Candida albicans, Gardnerella vaginalis, Trichomonas vaginalis,* or an imbalance of bacteria in the vagina.

Vaginosis can cause vaginitis. Vaginitis is inflammation of the vagina resulting in itching, burning, fishy-smelling discharge, painful intercourse, soreness, and redness.

Women with gynecologic infections have more than one infection in 55.2% of cases. HPV is the most common infection in 49.4%, followed by bacterial vaginosis in 33.5%.

Dr. Veena Singh and five medical colleagues at the Institute of Cytology and Preventative Oncology of Maulana Azad Medical College in New Delhi India published an article in the February 1995 issue of the *Obstetrics and Gynecology* journal. They described a study of 257 women and the various gynecologic infections found. HPV was found in 49.4%. Warts were seen in 2.7%. Bacterial vaginosis was detected in 33.5%. Antibodies to the herpes simplex virus were detected in 20.6%. And 55.2% of the women had two or more infections. In conclusion, Dr. Singh says:

> The specific finding of bleeding cervices was associated with HPV and bacterial vaginosis, hypertrophied cervices with *Chlamydia* and bacterial vaginosis, and unhealthy cervices with *Chlamydia* and HPV infections.

[Singh, V., et al. (1995). Clinical presentation of gynecologic infections among Indian women. *Obstet Gynecol. 1995 Feb; 85 (2): 215-9.* https://pubmed.ncbi. nlm.nih.gov/7824233/]

HPV infections and bacterial vaginosis infections have similar signs and symptoms. Bacterial vaginosis is more common among patients with HPV infections.

Dr. B. Sikstrom and four medical colleagues at the Institute of Clinical Bacteriology of Uppsala University in Uppsala Sweden published an article in the 1997 issue of the *Gynecologic and Obstetric Investigation* journal. Dr. Sikstrom found that 6.8% of the women had a cervical HPV infection. Bacterial vaginosis was more common among those with HPV. Vaginal discharge with a fishy odor, a positive amine test, and genital fissures correlated significantly with HPV. Symptoms of proctitis also correlated with HPV.

[Sikstrom, B., et al. (1997). Gynecological symptoms and vaginal wet smear findings in women with cervical human papillomavirus infection. *Gynecol Obstet Invest. 1997; 43 (1): 49-52.* https://pubmed.ncbi.nlm.nih.gov/ 9015700/]

Dr. P.A. Mardh and three medical colleagues at the Center of Sexually Transmitted Diseases of Uppsala University in Uppsala Sweden published an article in the November 1998 issue of the *International Journal of Gynaecology and Obstetrics*. The article compared the signs and symptoms of genital infections. The study included 996 healthy women. Dr. Mardh said:

When co-infections were excluded, *Chlamydial* infections, bacterial vaginosis, and cervical human papillomavirus infections were associated with a fishy malodor. Vaginal candidiasis showed characteristic symptoms and signs. Genital warts were associated with dysuria, general and lower abdominal pain.

[Mardh, P.A., et al. (1998). Symptoms and signs in single and mixed genital infections. *Int J Gynaecol Obstet. 1998 Nov; 63 (2): 145-52.* https://pubmed.ncbi. nlm.nih.gov/9856320/]

Subclinical HPV infections are associated with the symptoms of bacterial vaginosis.

"Subclinical" may refer to any disease that is not severe enough to cause the symptoms classically associated with that disease.

Doctors Anders Strand and Eva Rylander at the Department of Medicine of the University Hospital in Uppsala Sweden published an article in the October 1998 issue of the *Dermatology Clinics* journal describing subclinical and atypical manifestations of HPV. In this article, Dr. Strand noted:

Subclinical HPV infections, together with latent infections, are probably the most likely outcome after exposure to HPV. Subclinical infection is associated with symptoms such as burning, fissuring, and dyspareunia, or painful intercourse, in some patients. Recently, results have been presented showing a median duration of HPV infection of only 8 months, and after 24 months, only 9% of the women studied continued to be infected. This provides the possibility to reassure patients with HPV infection that it is most likely a transient infection, and one should not worry unduly.

[Strand, A., et al. (1998). Human papillomavirus. Subclinical and atypical manifestations. *Dermatol Clin. 1998 Oct; 16 (4): 817-22.* https://pubmed.ncbi.nlm.nih. gov/9891687/]

Bacterial vaginosis has a poor response to antimicrobial therapy. This would be expected since most cervical infections are viral and are frequently caused by HPV.

Dr. Venna Singh and five medical colleagues at the Institute of Cytology and Preventative Oncology of Marg in New Delhi India published an article in the April 1999 issue of the *Diagnostic Cytopathology* journal. Of 257 women, 207 had inflammatory cervical smears, of which 183 were infected with one or more genital tract infections. Bacterial vaginosis, *Chlamydia*, and HPV were each associated with inflammatory smears. In addition, significantly higher proportions of women with inflammatory smears had cervical ectopies and bleeding ectopies compared to noninflammatory smears. A cervical ectopy is a red and raw appearing area on the outer surface of the cervix. Dr. Singh found that most of the infections do not respond to antimicrobial therapy since they are viral in nature and frequently caused by HPV.

[Singh, V., et al. (1999). Biological behavior and etiology of inflammatory cervical smears. *Diagn Cytopathol. 1999 Apr; 20 (4): 199-202.* https://pubmed. ncbi.nlm.nih.gov/10204101/]

A strong association between bacterial vaginosis and HPV infection was found in a study of 6,372 women.

Dr. Evy Gillet and six medical colleagues at the International Centre for Reproductive Health of Ghent University in Ghent Belgium published an article in the January 2011 issue of the *BMC Infectious Diseases* journal. Dr. Gillet found:

Bacterial vaginosis (BV), an alteration of vaginal flora involving a decrease in *Lactobacilli* and predominance of anaerobic bacteria, is among the most common cause of vaginal complaints for women of childbearing age. The objective of this meta-analysis of published studies is to clarify and summarize published literature on the extent to which BV is associated with cervical HPV infection. Twelve eligible studies were selected to review the association between BV and HPV, including a total of 6,372 women. The pooled prevalence of BV was 32%. This meta-analysis of available literature resulted in a positive association between BV and uterine cervical HPV infection.

[Gillet, E., et al. (2011). Bacterial vaginosis is associated with uterine cervical human papillomavirus infection: a meta-analysis. *BMC Infect Dis. 2011 Jan 11; 11: 10.* https://pubmed.ncbi.nlm.nih.gov/21223574/]

Dr. Rodrigo Cesar Assis Caixeta at the Department of Pathology of the Federal University of Goiás in Goiânia Brazil, and six medical colleagues, published an article in the October 2015 issue of the *Diagnostic Cytopathology* journal. Dr. Caixeta reported HPV's association with bacterial vaginosis and said:

HPV, BV, and cervicitis were found in 44.2%, 41.0%, and 83.2% of cases, respectively. Cytological abnormalities were significantly associated with a finding of HPV and BV in the same woman, and also with a simultaneous finding of HPV, BV, and cervicitis.

[Caixeta, R.C.A., et al. (2015). Association between the human papillomavirus, bacterial vaginosis, and cervicitis and the detection of abnormalities in cervical smears from teenage girls and young women. *Diagn Cytopathol. 2015 Oct; 43 (10): 780-5.* https://pubmed. ncbi.nlm.nih.gov/26173042/]

Dr. L.T. Meng and five medical colleagues at the Department of Obstetrics and Gynecology of Xi'an Jiao-tong University in Xi'an China published an article in the October 2016 issue of the *Zhonghua Fu Chan Ke Za Zhi* journal. They examined HPV infection in bacterial vaginosis. Dr. Meng said:

142 cases of BV had 54 cases infected with HPV, 296 cases of intermediate type BV had 88 cases infected with HPV. The intensity of HPV infection was positively correlated with BV. BV and intermediate type BV positively correlate with HPV infection, especially for the high-risk HPV.

[Meng, L.T., et al. (2016). Relationship of HPV infection and BV, VVC, TV: a clinical study based on 1,261 cases of gynecologic outpatients. *Zhonghua Fu Chan Ke Za Zhi. 2016 Oct 25; 51 (10): 730-733.* https://pubmed. ncbi.nlm.nih.gov/27788738/]

A strong association between bacterial vaginosis and HPV infection was found in a study of 10,546 women.

Dr. Wissam Dahoud and four medical colleagues at the Department of Pathology of Case Western Reserve University School of Medicine in Cleveland Ohio published an article in the July 2019 issue of the *American Journal of Clinical Pathology*. These doctors examined bacterial vaginosis, HPV, and cervical dysplasia associations. Dr. Dahoud found bacterial vaginosis more common among patients with HPV infection. Dr. Dahoud said:

A retrospective study was performed on 10,546 cases. BV was present in 17.6% of cases. There was a significant association between BV, positive HPV infection, and high-grade SIL. We found there is a significant association between BV and SIL. BV is more common among patients with HPV infection.

[Dahoud, W., et al. (2019). Association of bacterial vaginosis and human papillomavirus infection with cervical squamous intraepithelial lesions. *Am J Clin Pathol. 2019 Jul 5; 152 (2): 185-189.* https://pubmed.ncbi.nlm.nih.gov/31065675/]

Bacterial vaginosis was related to HPV 51 and HPV 52 in a study of 2,000 women.

Dr. Wenyu Lin at the Department of Gynecology of Fujian Medical University in Fuzhou China, and five medical colleagues, published an article in the December 2021 issue of the *BMC Women's Health* journal. They examined the prevalence of HPV and bacterial vaginosis in young women. Dr. Lin concluded:

> The objective of this study was to assess the epidemiology of HPV combined with BV prevalence among Chinese women aged 20-35 years. A total of 2,000 sexually active women voluntarily enrolled in this study. The overall HPV infection rate in this population was 16.2%. In patients with cervical lesions, the BV prevalence rate was higher than in patients negative for intraepithelial lesions. BV was found to be related to HPV 51 and HPV 52 infections and cervical lesions.

[Lin, W., et al. (2021). The prevalence of human papillomavirus and bacterial vaginosis among young women in China: a cross-sectional study. *BMC Womens Health. 2021 Dec 9; 21 (1): 409.* https://pubmed.ncbi.nlm.nih.gov/34886845/]

These studies have demonstrated an association of HPV with vaginosis. It is worthwhile to have an HPV test performed in all cases of suspected HPV.

HPV-negative tests do not rule out an HPV infection because (1) less than 10% of the known 228 HPV types

are usually tested, and (2) the tests can yield false-negative results even for the few types tested. Therefore, treatment may be considered if HPV is suspected in the presence of HPV symptoms in the patient or the patient's partner.

Chapter 43
Vulvar Vestibulitis Syndrome

There is good evidence that vulvar vestibulitis syndrome, also known as VVS, can be caused by HPV.

Vulvar vestibulitis, a type of vulvodynia, affects many American women. Patients typically present with a history of intermittent or continuous, localized, vulvar pain and frequently cannot tolerate sexual intercourse, also known as dyspareunia.

HPV is one of the causes of vulvar vestibulitis syndrome.

Dr. M.L. Turner and Dr. S.C. Marinoff at the Department of Dermatology of George Washington University Medical School in Washington DC published an article in the June 1988 issue of the *Journal of Reproductive Medicine*. It discussed the association of HPV with vulvodynia and vulvar vestibulitis syndrome. Dr. Turner said:

> Seven women presenting with longstanding introital dyspareunia and burning in the vulvar area were demonstrated to harbor human papillomavirus. We propose that HPV infection is one of the causes of vulvodynia and the vulvar vestibulitis syndrome.

[Turner, M.L., and Marinoff, S.C. (1988). Association of human papillomavirus with vulvodynia and the vulvar vestibulitis syndrome. *J Reprod Med. 1988 Jun; 33 (6): 533-7.* https://pubmed.ncbi.nlm.nih.gov/2841460/]

HPV infections are found in 54% of women with severe vulvar vestibulitis syndrome versus approximately 13% in the general population.

Dr. Jacob Bornstein and six medical colleagues at the Department of Obstetrics and Gynecology of Carmel Medical Center in Haifa Israel published an article in the July 1996 issue of the *American Journal of Obstetrics and Gynecology*. They examined the evidence for a cause of vulvar vestibulitis syndrome. Among 86 women with severe VVS, 54% had HPV.

[Bornstein, J., et al. (1996). Polymerase chain reaction search for viral etiology of vulvar vestibulitis syndrome. *Am J Obstet Gynecol 1996 Jul; 175 (1): 139-44.* https://pubmed.ncbi.nlm.nih.gov/8694039/]

These studies have demonstrated an association of HPV with vulvar vestibulitis. It is worthwhile to have an HPV test performed in all cases of suspected HPV.

HPV-negative tests do not rule out an HPV infection because (1) less than 10% of the known 228 HPV types are usually tested, and (2) the tests can yield false-negative results even for the few types tested. Therefore, treatment may be considered if HPV is suspected in the presence of HPV symptoms in the patient or the patient's partner.

Chapter 44
Lichen Sclerosus

L ichen sclerosus is a skin lesion that begins as a small, bluish-white papule. Frequently, the coalescence of multiple papules produces a picture of diffuse whitish change over the entire vulva and peri-anal region. There is good evidence that lichen sclero-sus, also known as LS, can be caused by HPV.

HPV was detected in 70-80% of lichen sclerosus - a significantly higher percentage than approximately 13% found in the general population.

Dr. Rosa Monica Drut and three medical colleagues at the Department of Pathology of Hospital de Ninos in La Plata Argentina published an article in the March 1998 issue of the journal of *Pediatric Dermatology*. They presented findings of HPV in lichen sclerosus. Lichen sclerosus is a skin disease that may affect both sexes at all ages and at any site. Dr. Drut said that the results demonstrated the presence of HPV in roughly 70% of cases of lichen sclerosus.

[Drut, R.M., et al. (1998). Human papillomavirus is present in some cases of childhood penile lichen sclerosus: an in situ hybridization and SP-PCR study. *Pediatr Dermatol. Mar-Apr 1998; 15 (2): 85-90.* https://pubmed. ncbi.nlm.nih.gov/9572688/]

Dr. Anna K. Hald at the Aarhus University in Aarhus Denmark and Dr. Jan Blaakaer at the Department of Obstetrics and Gynaecology of Odense University Hospital in Odense Denmark published an article in the February 2018 issue of the *International Journal of Dermatology* about HPV and lichen sclerosus. Dr. Hald said:

Lichen sclerosus is a chronic inflammatory skin disease of unknown origin predominantly affecting the anogenital area that causes pruritus and pain and is associated with an increased risk of malignancy. In some cases, LS vanishes after the application of imiquimod, raising the question of whether human papillomavirus may have an etiopathogenic role in anogenital LS. Twenty-seven papers reported the prevalence of HPV in LS and LS associated with neoplasia. HPV was identified in up to 80% of all LS cases. The prevalence of HPV was higher among male patients with LS than among female patients. HPV 16 was the most prevalent, but the distribution indicates that even low-risk HPV can cause LS. Factors possibly underestimating the prevalence of HPV are a selective search for high-risk HPV, DNA destruction in fixed tissue, focally residing HPV, and possibly a clearing of HPV before the time of biopsy.

[Hald, A.K., and Blaakaer, J. (2018). The possible role of human papillomavirus infection in the development of lichen sclerosus. *Int J Dermatol. 2018 Feb; 57 (2): 139-146.* https://pubmed.ncbi.nlm.nih.gov/28737238/]

These studies have demonstrated an association of HPV with lichen sclerosus. It is worthwhile to have an HPV test performed in all cases of suspected HPV.

HPV-negative tests do not rule out an HPV infection because (1) less than 10% of the known 228 HPV types are usually tested, and (2) the tests can yield false-negative results even for the few types tested. Therefore, treatment may be considered if HPV is suspected in the presence of HPV symptoms in the patient or the patient's partner.

Chapter 45
Skin Tags and Various Skin Lesions

H PV has been found in various skin lesions. **HPV has been detected in skin tags, lichen sclerosus, epidermal cysts, and psoriatic plaques.**

Dr. Suzana Ljubojevic and Dr. Mihael Skerlev at the Department of Dermatology of the School of Medicine University in Zagreb Croatia published an article in the March 2014 issue of the *Clinics of Dermatology* journal. They discussed HPV-associated diseases. They point out that over 200 HPV types have been discovered, and each may be associated with various types of skin and mucosal lesions of the genital and non-genital regions. These include benign warts and cancer of the cervix, vulva, anus, and penis. Dr. Ljubojevic said: "HPV's have also been detected in skin tags, lichen sclerosus, seborrheic keratoses, actinic keratoses, epidermal cysts, psoriatic plaques, and plucked hairs."

[Ljubojevic, S., et al. (2014). HPV-associated diseases. *Clin Dermatol. Mar-Apr 2014; 32 (2): 227-34.* https://pubmed.ncbi.nlm.nih.gov/24559558/]

This study has demonstrated an association of HPV with various skin conditions. It is worthwhile to have an HPV test performed in all cases of suspected HPV.

HPV-negative tests do not rule out an HPV infection because (1) less than 10% of the known 228 HPV types are usually tested, and (2) the tests can yield false-negative results even for the few types tested. Therefore, treatment may be considered if HPV is suspected in the presence of HPV symptoms in the patient or the patient's partner.

Epilogue

This book presented the essential facts about HPV, Pap smears, cervical dysplasia, and warts. It included critical information about HPV diagnosis and treatment.

We evaluated various treatments of HPV, determined how to treat it effectively, and how best to develop immunity to it.

This book provided facts about these topics.

- HPV diagnosis, transmission, treatments, and immunity.
- Cervical dysplasia diagnosis and treatments.
- Warts diagnosis and treatments.

- HPV risks for infertility, miscarriages, pregnancy, and cervical cancer.
- Oral HPV, anal HPV, urethritis, and vaginosis.
- HPV risks for penile cancer and prostate disease.

We covered these seven Parts and topics.

Part I: Fundamentals of HPV and Cervical Dysplasia. The natural history of HPV, immunology of HPV, HPV types, HPV reinfection, and cervical cancer.

Part II: Diagnosis of HPV and Cervical Dysplasia. Pap smear screening, limitations of ASCUS Pap smears, self-sampling for HPV, degrees of cervical dysplasia, colposcopy and biopsy, and HPV false-negative results.

Part III: Transmission and Prevalence of HPV. HPV transmission in general, HPV transmission during childbirth, cervical dysplasia during pregnancy, and prevalence and public awareness of HPV.

Part IV: Treatment of Cervical Dysplasia. Medical treatments of trichloroacetic acid and 5-fluorouracil; surgical treatments of LEEP, cone biopsy, and cryotherapy; alternative treatments of beta-carotene, folic acid, vitamin C, indole-3-carbinol, AHCC, and Betamannan™; the value of *Aloe vera* and iodine as critical supports for the immune system to prevent and treat infections. The evidence showed that Beta-mannan™ is an effective alternative therapy for HPV, more effective than expected from the natural history of cervical dysplasia or warts.

Part V: Diagnosis and Treatment of Warts. Genital, plantar, palmar, flat, and common warts; medical, surgical, and alternative treatments; conditions that may be confused with warts such as pearly penile papules and molluscum contagiosum.

Part VI: Men and HPV. HPV-related diseases in men such as penile cancer, prostate disease, and prostate cancer.

Part VII: HPV-associated Conditions. Infertility, miscarriages, oral lesions, anal cancer, urethritis, vaginosis, vulvar vestibulitis syndrome, lichen sclerosus, and skin tags.

Afterword

Immunity to HPV is acquired frequently.

Immunity to HPV must specify a particular HPV type - one of the 228 currently identified. If a person tests positive for a particular type or types, but later tests negative for them, then that person has achieved immunity for those particular types, assuming the test result is not a false-negative result.

HPV-negative tests do not rule out an HPV infection because (1) less than 10% of the known 228 HPV types are usually tested, and (2) the tests can yield false-negative results even for the few types tested. Therefore, treatment may be considered if HPV is suspected in the presence of HPV symptoms in the patient or the patient's partner.

Afterword

If you found this book helpful, I would appreciate a favorable review on Amazon®.

C.W. Willington

Bibliography

Abraham, G.E. and Brownstein, D. (2005). *Townsend Letter: A rebuttal of Dr. Gaby's editorial on iodine.* Townsend Letter: Port Townsend, Washington. Retrieved 3 July 2022 https://www.townsendletter. com/Oct2005/gabyrebuttal1005.htm

Aceves, C., et al. (2013). The extrathyronine actions of iodine as antioxidant, apoptotic, and differentiation factor in various tissues. *Thyroid. 2013 Aug; 23 (8): 938–946.* https://www.ncbi. nlm.nih.gov/pmc/articles/PMC3752513/

Agarwal, O.P. (1985). Prevention of atheromatous heart disease. *Angiology. 1985 Aug; 36 (8): 485-92.* https://www.desertharvest. com/physicians/documents/DH155.pdf https://bit.ly/angiologys tudy https://pubmed.ncbi.nlm.nih.gov/2864002/

Agliano, A.M., et al. (1994). Detection of human papillomavirus type 16 DNA sequences in paraffin-embedded tissues from the female urinary tract. *Urol Int. 1994; 52 (4): 208-12.* https://pubmed.ncbi. nlm.nih.gov/8030168/

Aldahan, A.S., et al. (2016). Diagnosis and management of pearly penile papules. *Am J Mens Health. 2018 May; 12 (3): 624-627.* https://www.ncbi.nlm.nih.gov/pmc/articles/PMC5987947/

Alinejad-Mofrad, S., et al. (2015). Improvement of glucose and lipid profile status with *Aloe vera* in pre-diabetic subjects: a random-ized controlled-trial. *J Diabetes Metab Disord. 2015 Apr 9; 14: 22.* https://pubmed.ncbi.nlm.nih.gov/25883909/

Anguiano, B., et al. (2011). Iodine in mammary and prostate patholo-gies. *Current Chemical Biology, Volume 5, Number 3, 2011, pp. 177-182 (6).* https://www.ingentaconnect.com/content/ben/ccb/2011/ 00000005/00000003/art00005

Aranda, N., et al. (2013). Uptake and anti-tumoral effects of iodine and 6-iodolactone in differentiated and undifferentiated human prostate cancer cell lines. *Prostate. 2013 Jan; 73 (1): 31-41.* https://pubmed.ncbi.nlm.nih.gov/22576883/

Arthur, J.R., et al. (1999). The interactions between selenium and iodine deficiencies in man and animals. *Nutr Res Rev. 1999 Jun; 12 (1): 55-73.* https://pubmed.ncbi.nlm.nih.gov/19087446/

Auborn, K.J. (2006). Can indole-3-carbinol-induced changes in cervical intraepithelial neoplasia be extrapolated to other food components? *J Nutr 2006 Oct; 136 (10): 2676S-8S.* https://pubmed.ncbi.nlm.nih.gov/16988146/

Baldauf, J.J., et al. (1997). Consequences and treatment of cervical stenoses after laser conization or loop electrosurgical excision. *J Gynecol Obstet Biol Reprod (Paris). 1997; 26 (1): 64-70.* https://pubmed.ncbi.nlm.nih.gov/9091546/

Baldwin, S.B., et al. (2003). Human papillomavirus infection in men attending a sexually transmitted disease clinic. *J Infect Dis. 2003 Apr 1; 187 (7): 1064-70.* https://pubmed.ncbi.nlm.nih.gov/12660920/

Barchitta, M. (2020). Dietary antioxidant intake and human papillomavirus infection: evidence from a cross-sectional study in Italy. *Nutrients. 2020 May; 12 (5): 1384.* https://pubmed.ncbi.nlm.nih.gov/32408636/

Barzon, L., et al. (2010). Distribution of human papillomavirus types in the anogenital tract of females and males. *J Med Virol. 2010 Aug; 82 (8): 1424-30.* https://pubmed.ncbi.nlm.nih.gov/20572068/

Bell, M.C., et al. (2000). Placebo-controlled trial of indole-3-carbinol in the treatment of CIN. *Gynecol Oncol. 2000 Aug; 78 (2): 123-9.* https://pubmed.ncbi.nlm.nih.gov/10926790/

Bennett, M. (2022). *The Olive Leaf: Testimonials.* The Olive Leaf: Atlanta, Georgia. Retrieved 3 July 2022 https://theoliveleaf.com/testimonials/

Bilal, M.Y., et al. (2017). A role for iodide and thyroglobulin in modulating the function of human immune cells. *Front Immunol. 2017 Nov 15; 8: 1573.* https://pubmed.ncbi.nlm.nih.gov/29187856/

Bober, L., et al. (2019). Influence of human papillomavirus (HPV) infection on early pregnancy. *Ginekol Pol. 2019; 90 (2): 72-75.* https://pubmed.ncbi.nlm.nih.gov/30860272/

Boels, David, et al. (2022). Shiitake dermatitis: experience of the Poison Control Centre Network in France from 2014 to 2019. *Clin Toxicol (Phila). 2022 Apr 11; 1-6.* https://pubmed.ncbi.nlm.nih.gov/35404185/

Bornstein, J., et al. (1996). Polymerase chain reaction search for viral etiology of vulvar vestibulitis syndrome. *Am J Obstet Gynecol 1996 Jul; 175 (1): 139-44.* https://pubmed.ncbi.nlm.nih.gov/8694039/

Bougma, K., et al. (2013). Iodine and mental development of children 5 years old and under: a systematic review and meta-analysis. *Nutrients. 2013 Apr 22; 5 (4): 1384-416.* https://pubmed.ncbi.nlm.nih.gov/23609774/

Boxman, I.L.A., et al. (1999). Detection of human papillomavirus types 6 and 11 in pubic and perianal hair from patients with genital warts. *J Clin Microbiol. 1999 Jul; 37 (7): 2270-3.* https://pubmed.ncbi.nlm.nih.gov/10364596/

Boyages, S.C., et al. (1989). Iodine deficiency impairs intellectual and neuromotor development in apparently normal persons. A study of rural inhabitants of north-central China. *Med J Aust. 1989 Jun 19; 150 (12): 676-82.* https://pubmed.ncbi.nlm.nih.gov/2733614/

Braaten, K.P., et al. (2008). Human Papillomavirus (HPV), HPV-Related Disease, and the HPV Vaccine. *Rev Obstet Gynecol. 2008 Winter; 1 (1): 2–10.* https://www.ncbi.nlm.nih.gov/pmc/articles/PMC2492590/

Brouwer, A.F., et al. (2022). Incidence and clearance of oral and cervicogenital HPV infection: longitudinal analysis of the MHOC cohort study. *BMJ Open. 2022 Jan 3; 12 (1): e056502.* https://pubmed.ncbi.nlm.nih.gov/34980629/

Brownstein, D. (2009). *Iodine: Why You Need It, Why You Can't Live*

Bibliography

Without It (4th Edition). West Bloomfield, Michigan: Medical Alternatives Press.

Bruggink, S.C., et al. (2013). Natural course of cutaneous warts among primary school children: a prospective cohort study. *Ann Fam Med. 2013 Sep; 11 (5): 437–441.* https://pubmed.ncbi.nlm.nih.gov/24019275/

Bruno, M.T., et al. (2021). Progression of CIN-1/LSIL HPV persistent of the cervix: actual progression or CIN-3 coexistence. *Infect Dis Obstet Gynecol. 2021 Mar 9; 2021: 6627531,* https://pubmed.ncbi.nlm.nih.gov/33776406/

Burd, E.M. (2003). Human papillomavirus and cervical cancer. *Clin Microbiol Rev. 2003 Jan; 16 (1): 1–17.* https://www.ncbi.nlm.nih.gov/pmc/articles/PMC145302/

Caixeta, R.C.A., et al. (2015). Association between the human papillomavirus, bacterial vaginosis, and cervicitis and the detection of abnormalities in cervical smears from teenage girls and young women. *Diagn Cytopathol. 2015 Oct; 43 (10): 780-5.* https://pubmed.ncbi.nlm.nih.gov/26173042/

Cann, S.A., et al. (2000). Hypothesis: iodine, selenium and the development of breast cancer. *Cancer Causes Control. 2000 Feb; 11 (2): 121-7.* https://pubmed.ncbi.nlm.nih.gov/10710195/

Cellini, L., et al. (2014). In vitro activity of *Aloe vera* inner gel against *Helicobacter pylori* strains. *Lett Appl Microbiol. 2014 Jul; 59 (1): 43-8.* https://pubmed.ncbi.nlm.nih.gov/24597562/

Cheah, P.L., et al. (1998). Biology and pathological associations of the human papillomaviruses: a review. *Malays J Pathol. 1998 Jun; 20 (1): 1-10.* https://pubmed.ncbi.nlm.nih.gov/10879257/

Chiarini, F., et al. (1998). Simultaneous detection of HPV and other sexually transmitted agents in chronic urethritis. *Minerva Urol Nefrol. 1998 Dec; 50 (4): 225-31.* https://pubmed.ncbi.nlm.nih.gov/9973807/

Cooper, D.B., et al. (2021). Conization of cervix. Treasure Island, Florida: *StatPearls Publishing. December 2021.* https://www.ncbi.nlm.nih.gov/books/NBK441845/

Cowan, D. (2010). Oral *Aloe vera* as a treatment for osteoarthritis: a summary. *Br J Community Nurs. 2010 Jun; 15 (6): 280-2.* https://pubmed.ncbi.nlm.nih.gov/20679979/

Cubie, H.A., et al. (1998). Presence of antibodies to human papillomavirus virus-like particles (VLPs) in 11-13-year-old schoolgirls. *J Med Virol. 1998 Nov; 56 (3): 210-6.* https://pubmed.ncbi.nlm.nih.gov/9783687/

Cui, M., et al. (2014). Clinical performance of Roche Cobas 4800 HPV test. *J Clin Microbiol. 2014 Jun; 52 (6): 2210–2211.* https://www.ncbi.nlm.nih.gov/pmc/articles/PMC4042746/

Cupp, M.R., et al. (1995). The detection of human papillomavirus deoxyribonucleic acid in intraepithelial, in situ, verrucous and invasive carcinoma of the penis. *J Urol. 1995 Sep; 154 (3): 1024-9.* https://pubmed.ncbi.nlm.nih.gov/7637047/

D'Alessandro, P., et al. (2018). Loop electrosurgical excision procedure versus cryotherapy in the treatment of cervical intraepithelial-neoplasia: A systematic review and meta-analysis of randomized controlled trials. *Gynecol Minim Invasive Ther. 2018 Oct-Dec; 7 (4): 145–151.* https://pubmed.ncbi.nlm.nih.gov/30306032/

Dahoud, W., et al. (2019). Association of bacterial vaginosis and human papillomavirus infection with cervical squamous intraepithelial lesions. *Am J Clin Pathol. 2019 Jul 5; 152 (2): 185-189.* https://pubmed.ncbi.nlm.nih.gov/31065675/

Damani, M.R., et al. (2015). Treatment of ocular surface squamous neoplasia with topical *Aloe vera* drops. *Cornea. 2015 Jan; 34 (1): 87-9.* https://pubmed.ncbi.nlm.nih.gov/25393094/

de Gaia, Zayna. (2013). *Thank You for HPV, pp. 64-65.*

DiNicolantonio, J.J., et al. (2018). Subclinical magnesium deficiency: a principal driver of cardiovascular disease and a public health

crisis. *Open Heart. 2018; 5 (1): e000668.* https://www.ncbi.nlm.
nih.gov/pmc/articles/PMC5786912/

Drut, R.M., et al. (1998). Human papillomavirus is present in some
cases of childhood penile lichen sclerosus: an in situ hybridization and SP-PCR study. *Pediatr Dermatol. Mar-Apr 1998; 15 (2):
85-90.* https://pubmed.ncbi.nlm.nih.gov/9572688/

Earth Clinic LLC. (2022). *Genital HPV Remedies: Aloe with Beta-
mannan™.* Earth Clinic LLC: Norwalk, Connecticut. Retrieved 3
July ???? https://www.earthclinic.com/cures/natural-hpv-treat-
ment.html#bm

Edwards, L., et al. (1998.) Self-administered topical 5% imiquimod
cream for external anogenital warts. HPV Study Group. Human
PapillomaVirus. *Arch Dermatol. 1998 Jan; 134 (1): 25-30.* https://
pubmed.ncbi.nlm.nih.gov/9449906/

Eggersmann, T.K., et al. (2019). Prevalence of oral HPV infection in
cervical HPV-positive women and their sexual partners. *Arch
Gynecol Obstet. 2019 Jun; 299 (6): 1659-1665.* https://pubmed.ncbi.
nlm.nih.gov/30953186/

Elfgren, K., et al. (1996). Conization for cervical intraepithelial
neoplasia is followed by disappearance of human papillomavirus
deoxyribonucleic acid and a decline in serum and cervical mucus
antibodies against human papillomavirus antigens. *Am J Obstet
Gynecol. 1996 Mar; 174 (3): 937-42.* https://pubmed.ncbi.nlm.nih.
gov/8633673/

Eskin, B.A. (1983). Iodine and breast cancer: 1982 update. *Biol Trace
Elem Res. 1983 Aug; 5 (4-5): 399-412.* https://pubmed.ncbi.nlm.
nih.gov/24263577/

Ferenczy, A., et al. (1991). Pearly penile papules: absence of human
papillomavirus DNA by the polymerase chain reaction. *Obstet
Gynecol. 1991 Jul; 78 (1): 118-22.* https://pubmed.ncbi.nlm.nih.gov/
2047052/

Fetters, M.D., et al. (1996). Effectiveness of vaginal Papanicolaou
smear screening after total hysterectomy for benign disease.

JAMA. 1996 Mar 27; 275 (12): 940-7. https://pubmed.ncbi.nlm.nih.gov/8598623/

Foresta, C., et al. (2015). HPV-DNA sperm infection and infertility: from a systematic literature review to a possible clinical management proposal. *Andrology. 2015 Mar; 3 (2): 163-73.* https://pubmed.ncbi.nlm.nih.gov/25270519/

Frega, A., et al. (2007). Clinical management and follow-up of squamous intraepithelial cervical lesions during pregnancy and postpartum. *Anticancer Res. Jul-Aug 2007; 27 (4C): 2743-6.* https://pubmed.ncbi.nlm.nih.gov/17695441/

Garcia-Oreja, S., et al. (2021). Topical treatment for plantar warts: A systematic review. *Dermatol Ther. 2021 Jan; 34 (1): e14621.* https://pubmed.ncbi.nlm.nih.gov/33263934/

Ghent, W.R., et al. (1993). Iodine replacement in fibrocystic disease of the breast. *Can J Surg. 1993 Oct; 36 (5): 453-60.* https://pubmed.ncbi.nlm.nih.gov/8221402/

Gilham, C., et al. (2019). HPV testing compared with routine cytology in cervical screening: long-term follow-up of ARTISTIC RCT. *Health Technol Assess. 2019 Jun; 23 (28): 1-44.* https://pubmed.ncbi.nlm.nih.gov/31219027/

Gillet, E., et al. (2011). Bacterial vaginosis is associated with uterine cervical human papillomavirus infection: a meta-analysis. *BMC Infect Dis. 2011 Jan 11; 11: 10.* https://pubmed.ncbi.nlm.nih.gov/21223574/

Giuliano, A.R., et al. (1998). Can cervical dysplasia and cancer be prevented with nutrients? *Nutr Rev. 1998 Jan; 56 (1 Pt 1): 9-16.* https://pubmed.ncbi.nlm.nih.gov/9481113/

Glickman, J. (2022). *Beta-mannan™.* Beta-mannan™: Austin, Texas. Retrieved 3 July 2022 https://beta-mannan.com

Gorini, F., et al. (2021). Selenium: An element of life essential for thyroid function. *Molecules. 2021 Nov 23; 26 (23): 7084.* https://pubmed.ncbi.nlm.nih.gov/34885664/

Grenko, R.T., et al. (2000). Variance in the interpretation of cervical biopsy specimens obtained for atypical squamous cells of unde-termined significance. *Am J Clin Pathol. 2000 Nov; 114 (5): 735-40.* https://pubmed.ncbi.nlm.nih.gov/11068547/

Guo, X., et al. (2019). *Aloe vera:* A review of toxicity and adverse clin-ical effects. *J Environ Sci Health Rev. 2016 Apr 2; 34 (2): 77–96.* https://www.ncbi.nlm.nih.gov/pmc/articles/PMC6349368/

Hald, A.K., and Blaakaer, J. (2018). The possible role of human papil-lomavirus infection in the development of lichen sclerosus. *Int J Dermatol. 2018 Feb; 57 (2): 139-146.* https://pubmed.ncbi.nlm.nih.gov/28737238/

Hamza, R.T., et al. (2013). Iodine deficiency in Egyptian autistic chil-dren and their mothers: relation to disease severity. *Arch Med Res. 2013 Oct; 44 (7): 555-61.* https://pubmed.ncbi.nlm.nih.gov/24120386/

Harvard T.H. Chan Medical School of Public Health. (2022). *Nutrition and Immunity.* Harvard T.H. Chan Medical School of Public Health: Boston, Massachusetts. Retrieved 3 July 2022 https://www.hsph.harvard.edu/nutritionsource/nutrition-and-immunity/

Hashiguchi, M., et al. (2017). Effect of *Aloe*-emodin on the prolifera-tion and apoptosis of human synovial MH7A cells; a comparison with methotrexate. *Mol Med Rep. 2017 Jun; 15 (6): 4398-4404.* https://pubmed.ncbi.nlm.nih.gov/28487948/

Heideman, D.A.M., et al. (2013). The Aptima HPV assay fulfills the cross-sectional clinical and reproducibility criteria of international guidelines for human papillomavirus test require-ments for cervical screening. *J Clin Microbiol. 2013 Nov; 51 (11): 3653–3657.* https://www.ncbi.nlm.nih.gov/pmc/articles/PMC3889747/

Hellsten, C., et al. (2021). Equal prevalence of severe cervical dysplasia by HPV self-sampling and by midwife-collected samples for primary HPV screening: a randomized controlled trial. *Eur J Cancer Prev. 2021 Jul 1; 30 (4): 334-340.* https://pubmed.ncbi.nlm.nih.gov/34010238/

Hemmingsson, E. (1982). Outcome of third-trimester pregnancies after cryotherapy of the uterine cervix. *Br J Obstet Gynaecol. 1982 Aug; 89 (8): 675-7.* https://pubmed.ncbi.nlm.nih.gov/7104260/

Hermonat, P.L., et al. (1997). Human papillomavirus is more prevalent in first trimester spontaneously aborted specimens. *Virus Genes. 1997; 14 (1): 13-7.* https://pubmed.ncbi.nlm.nih.gov/9208451/

Hermonat, P.L., et al. (1998). Trophoblasts are the preferential target for human papillomavirus infection in spontaneously aborted. *Hum Pathol. 1998 Feb; 29 (2): 170-4.* https://pubmed.ncbi.nlm.nih.gov/9490277/

Husseinzadeh, N., et al. (1994). Subclinical cervicovaginal human papillomavirus infections associated with cervical condylomata and dysplasia. Treatment outcomes. *The Journal of Reproductive Medicine, 01 Oct 1994, 39 (10): 777-780.* https://pubmed.ncbi.nlm.nih.gov/7837123/

Icahn School of Medicine at Mount Sinai. (2022). *Mount Sinai.* Icahn School of Medicine at Mount Sinai: New York, New York. Retrieved 3 July 2022 https://www.mountsinai.org/profiles/charles-j-ascher-walsh

Ikeno, Y., et al. (2002). The influence of long-term *Aloe vera* ingestion on age-related disease in male Fischer 344 rats. *Phytother Res. 2002 Dec; 16 (8): 712-8.* https://pubmed.ncbi.nlm.nih.gov/12458471/

Im, S., et al. (2016). Prevention of azoxymethane/dextran sodium sulfate-induced mouse colon carcinogenesis by processed *Aloe vera* gel. *Int Immunopharmacol. 2016 Nov; 40: 428-435.* https://pubmed.ncbi.nlm.nih.gov/27697726/

Inthasorn, P., et al. (2021). Prevalence of abnormal anal cytology in women with abnormal cervical cytology. *Asian Pac J Cancer Prev.*

2021 Jul 1; 22 (7): 2165-2169. https://pubmed.ncbi.nlm.nih.gov/34319039/

Ittermann, T., et al. (2020). Standardized map of iodine status in Europe. *Thyroid. 2020 Sep; 30 (9): 1346-1354.* https://pubmed.ncbi.nlm.nih.gov/32460688/

J. Crow Co. (2022). *J. Crow's Marketplace.* J. Crow Co: New Ipswich, New Hampshire. Retrieved 3 July 2022 https://www.jcrowsmarketplace.com/

Jain, O., et al. (2016). Antibacterial effect of *Aloe vera* gel against oral pathogens: An in-vitro study. *J Clin Diagn Res. 2016 Nov; 10 (11): ZC41-ZC44.* https://pubmed.ncbi.nlm.nih.gov/28050502/

Jaworek, H., et al. (2019). Pitfalls of commercially available HPV tests in HPV 68a detection. *PLoS One. 2019 Aug 5; 14 (8): e0220373.* https://pubmed.ncbi.nlm.nih.gov/31381580/

Jee, B., et al. (2021). Immunology of HPV-mediated cervical cancer: current understanding. *Int Rev Immunol. 2021; 40 (5): 359-378.* https://pubmed.ncbi.nlm.nih.gov/32853049/

Jung, J.M., et al. (2020). Topically applied treatments for external genital warts in non-immunocompromised patients: a systematic review and network meta-analysis. *Br J Dermatol. 2020 Jul; 183 (1): 24-36.* https://pubmed.ncbi.nlm.nih.gov/31675442/

Kargar, S., et al. (2017). Urinary iodine concentrations in cancer patients. *Asian Pac J Cancer Prev. 2017 Mar 1; 18 (3): 819-821.* https://www.ncbi.nlm.nih.gov/pmc/articles/PMC5464505/

Karim, B., et al. (2014). Effect of *Aloe vera* mouthwash on periodontal health: triple blind randomized control trial. *Oral Health Dent Manag. 2014 Mar; 13 (1): 14-9.* https://pubmed.ncbi.nlm.nih.gov/24603910/

Kayes, L., et al. (2022). A review of current knowledge about the importance of iodine among women of childbearing age and healthcare professionals. *J Nutr Sci. 2022 Jul 8; 11: e56.* https://pubmed.ncbi.nlm.nih.gov/35836700/

Khieu, M., et al. (2022). High-grade squamous intraepithelial lesion.

Bibliography

Treasure Island, Florida: *StatPearls Publishing. January 5, 2022.* https://www.ncbi.nlm.nih.gov/books/NBK430728/

Kieliszek, M. (2019). Selenium–fascinating microelement, properties and sources in food. *Molecules. 2019 Apr; 24 (7): 1298.* https://www.ncbi.nlm.nih.gov/pmc/articles/PMC6480557/

Kilkenny, M., et al. (1998). The prevalence of common skin conditions in Australian school students: Common, plane and plantar viral warts. *Br J Dermatol. 1998 May; 138 (5): 840-5.* https://pubmed.ncbi.nlm.nih.gov/9666831/

Kolben, T.M., et al. (2017). Short interval between two Pap smears: effect on the result of the second smear? A prospective randomized trial. *Arch Gynecol Obstet. 2017 Jun; 295 (6): 1427-1433.* https://pubmed.ncbi.nlm.nih.gov/28405743/

Koshiol, J., et al. (2009). Knowledge of human papillomavirus. *J Health Commun. 2009 Jun; 14 (4): 331–345.* https://www.ncbi.nlm.nih.gov/pmc/articles/PMC2768561/

Koul, A., et al. (2015). *Aloe vera* affects changes induced in pulmonary tissue of mice caused by cigarette smoke inhalation. *Environ Toxicol. 2015 Sep; 30 (9): 999-1013.* https://pubmed.ncbi.nlm.nih.gov/24615921/

Kreimer, A.R., et al. (2013). Incidence and clearance of oral human papillomavirus infection in men: the HIM cohort study. *Lancet. 2013 Sep 7; 382 (9895): 877–887.* https://www.ncbi.nlm.nih.gov/pmc/articles/PMC3904652/

Kumar, R., et al. (2019). Therapeutic potential of *Aloe vera* - A miracle gift of nature. *Phytomedicine. 2019 Jul; 60: 152996.* https://pubmed.ncbi.nlm.nih.gov/31272819/

Kvicala, J., et al. (2003). Effect of iodine and selenium upon thyroid function. *Cent Eur J Public Health. 2003 Jun; 11 (2): 107-13.* https://pubmed.ncbi.nlm.nih.gov/12884559/

Kyrgiou, M., et al. (2016). Adverse obstetric outcomes after local treatment for cervical pre-invasive and early invasive disease according to cone depth: systematic review and meta-analysis.

Bibliography

BMJ. *2016; 354: i3633.* https://pubmed.ncbi.nlm.nih.gov/27469988/

Langmead, L., et al. (2004). Anti-inflammatory effects of *Aloe vera* gel in human colorectal mucosa in vitro. *Aliment Pharmacol Ther.* *2004 Mar 1; 19 (5): 521-7.* https://pubmed.ncbi.nlm.nih.gov/14987320/

Langmead, L., et al. (2004). Randomized, double-blind, placebo-controlled trial of oral *Aloe vera* gel for active ulcerative colitis. *Aliment Pharmacol Ther. 2004 Apr 1; 19 (7): 739 47.* https://pubmed.ncbi.nlm.nih.gov/15043514/

Lantsman, T., et al. (2020). Association between cervical dysplasia and adverse pregnancy outcomes. *Am J Perinatol. 2020 Jul; 37 (9): 947-954.* https://pubmed.ncbi.nlm.nih.gov/31167238/

Leaf Group Ltd. (2022). *eHow: How to take Beta-mannan™.* Leaf Group Ltd: Santa Monica California. Retrieved 3 July 2022 https://www.ehow.co.uk/how_8574055_beta-mannan.html

Lee, D., et al. (2018). Polysaccharide isolated from *Aloe vera* gel suppresses ovalbumin-induced food allergy through inhibition of Th2 immunity in mice. *Biomed Pharmacother. 2018 May; 101: 201-210.* https://pubmed.ncbi.nlm.nih.gov/29494957/

Lee, Y., et al. (2016). Modified *Aloe* polysaccharide restores chronic stress-induced immunosuppression in mice. *Int J Mol Sci. 2016 Oct; 17 (10): 1660.* https://www.ncbi.nlm.nih.gov/pmc/articles/PMC5085693/

Leslie, S.W., et al. (2022). Genital Warts. Treasure Island, Florida: *StatPearls Publishing. February 14, 2022.* https://www.ncbi.nlm.nih.gov/books/NBK441884/

Leung, A.K.C., et al. (2017). Molluscum contagiosum: an update. *Recent Pat Inflamm Allergy Drug Discov. 2017; 11 (1): 22-31.* https://pubmed.ncbi.nlm.nih.gov/28521677/

Lewis, R.M., et al. (2021). Estimated prevalence and incidence of disease-associated human papillomavirus types among 15-59 year-olds in the United States. *Sex Transm Dis. 2021 Apr 1; 48 (4): 273-277.* https://pubmed.ncbi.nlm.nih.gov/33492097/

Lin, W., et al. (2021). The prevalence of human papillomavirus and bacterial vaginosis among young women in China: a cross-sectional study. *BMC Womens Health. 2021 Dec 9; 21 (1): 409.* https://pubmed.ncbi.nlm.nih.gov/34886845/

Liota, E., et al. (2000). Imiquimod therapy for molluscum contagiosum. *J Cutan Med Surg. 2000 Apr; 4 (2): 76-82.* https://pubmed.ncbi.nlm.nih.gov/11179929/

Liu, Y., et al. (2022). Diagnostic value of colposcopy in patients with cytology-negative and HR-HPV-positive cervical lesions. *Arch Gynecol Obstet. 2022 Mar 23.* https://pubmed.ncbi.nlm.nih.gov/35320389/

Livasy, C.A., et al. (1999). Predictors of recurrent dysplasia after a cervical loop electrocautery excision procedure for CIN-3: a study of margin, endocervical gland, and quadrant involvement. *Mod Pathol. 1999 Mar; 12 (3): 233-8.* https://pubmed.ncbi.nlm.nih.gov/10102607/

Ljubojevic, S., et al. (2014). HPV-associated diseases. *Clin Dermatol. Mar-Apr 2014; 32 (2): 227-34.* https://pubmed.ncbi.nlm.nih.gov/24559558/

Loudwolf. (2022). *Loudwolf Industrial and Scientific Company.* Loudwolf: Dublin, California. Retrieved 3 July 2022 https://www.loudwolf.com/

Macios, A., et al. (2022). False-negative results in cervical cancer screening - risks, reasons, and implications for clinical practice and public health. *Diagnostics (Basel). 2022 Jun 20; 12 (6): 1508.* https://pubmed.ncbi.nlm.nih.gov/35741319/

Mackerras, D., et al. (1999). Randomized double-blind trial of beta-carotene and vitamin C in women with minor cervical abnormalities. *Br J Cancer. 1999 Mar; 79 (9-10): 1448–1453.* https://pubmed.ncbi.nlm.nih.gov/10188889/

Mardh, P.A., et al. (1998). Symptoms and signs in single and mixed genital infections. *Int J Gynaecol Obstet. 1998 Nov; 63 (2): 145-52.* https://pubmed.ncbi.nlm.nih.gov/9856320/

Mayer, C., et al. (2022). Abnormal Papanicolaou Smear. Treasure Island, Florida: *StatPearls Publishing. January 7, 2022.* https://www.ncbi.nlm.nih.gov/books/NBK560850/

McLachlin, C.M. (2000). Human papillomavirus in cervical neoplasia: role, risk factors, and implications. *Clin Lab Med 2000 Jun; 20 (2): 257-70.* https://pubmed.ncbi.nlm.nih.gov/10863640/

McNicol, P.J., et al. (1990). Detection of human papillomavirus DNA in prostate gland tissue by using the polymerase chain reaction amplification assay. *J Clin Microbiol. 1990 Mar; 28 (3): 409-12.* https://pubmed.ncbi.nlm.nih.gov/1691205/

Meng, L.T., et al. (2016). Relationship of HPV infection and BV, VVC, TV: a clinical study based on 1,261 cases of gynecologic outpatients. *Zhonghua Fu Chan Ke Za Zhi. 2016 Oct 25; 51 (10): 730-733.* https://pubmed.ncbi.nlm.nih.gov/27788738/

Metro, D., et al. (2018). Marked improvement of thyroid function and autoimmunity by *Aloe barbadensis miller* juice was shown in patients with subclinical hypothyroidism. *J Clin Transl Endocrinol. 2018 Mar; 11: 18–25.* https://www.ncbi.nlm.nih.gov/pmc/articles/PMC5842288/

Miles, E.A., et al. (2022). Iodine status in pregnant women and infants in Finland. *Eur J Nutr. 2022 Mar 19.* https://pubmed.ncbi.nlm.nih.gov/35305119/

Miller, D.W. (2006). Extra-thyroidal benefits of iodine. *Journal of American Physicians and Surgeons, Volume 11, Number 4, Winter 2006.* https://www.jpands.org/jpands1104.htm https://www.ign.org/cm_data/2006_Miller_Extrathyroidal_Benefits_of_Iodine.pdf

Mirshafiey, A., et al. (2010). Therapeutic approach by *Aloe vera* in experimental model of multiple sclerosis. *Immunopharmacology and Immunotoxicology. 2010 Sep; 32 (3): 410-5.* https://pubmed.ncbi.nlm.nih.gov/20233107/

Molnar, I., et al. (1998). Iodine deficiency in cardiovascular diseases.

Orv Hetil. 1998 Aug 30; 139 (35): 2071-3. https://pubmed.ncbi.nlm.nih.gov/9755626/

Monti, M., et al. (2021). Relationship between cervical excisional treatment for cervical intraepithelial neoplasia and obstetrical outcome. *Minerva Obstet Gynecol. 2021 Apr; 73 (2): 233-246.* https://pubmed.ncbi.nlm.nih.gov/33140628/

Moraczewski, T. (2012). *The Center for Natural and Integrative Medicine: HPV and Cervical Dysplasia – Alternatives to Conventional Therapy.* The Center for Natural and Integrative Medicine: Orlando, Florida. Retrieved 3 July 2022 https://drkalidas.com/uncategorized/hpv-cervical-dysplasia-alternatives-to-conventional-therapy/

Moriyama, M., et al. (2016). Beneficial effects of the genus *Aloe* on wound healing, cell proliferation, and differentiation of epidermal keratinocytes. *PLoS One. 2016; 11 (10): e0164799.* https://www.ncbi.nlm.nih.gov/pmc/articles/PMC5063354/

Moscicki, A.B., et al. (1998). The natural history of human papillomavirus infection as measured by repeated DNA testing in adolescents and young women. *J Pediatr. 1998 Feb; 132 (2): 277-84.* https://pubmed.ncbi.nlm.nih.gov/9506641/

Moscicki, A.B., et al. (1999). Risk factors for abnormal anal cytology in young heterosexual women. *Cancer Epidemiol Biomarkers Prev. 1999 Feb; 8 (2): 173-8.* https://pubmed.ncbi.nlm.nih.gov/10067816/

Moscicki, A.B., et al. (2004). Regression of low-grade squamous intra-epithelial lesions in young women. *Lancet. 2004 Nov 6-12; 364 (9446): 1678-83.* https://pubmed.ncbi.nlm.nih.gov/15530628/

Moscicki, A.B., et al. (2014). Natural history of anal human papillomavirus infection in heterosexual women and risks associated with persistence. *Clin Infect Dis. 2014 Mar; 58 (6): 804-11.* https://pubmed.ncbi.nlm.nih.gov/24368624/

Moyret-Lalle, C., et al. (1995). Ras, p53 and HPV status in benign and malignant prostate tumors. *Int J Cancer. 1995 Apr 21; 64 (2): 124-9.* https://pubmed.ncbi.nlm.nih.gov/7542226/

Mulki, A.K., et al. (2021). Human papillomavirus self-sampling performance in low- and middle-income countries. *BMC Women's Health. 2021 Jan 6; 21 (1): 12.* https://pubmed.ncbi.nlm.nih.gov/33407355/

Munoz, N. (2000). Human papillomavirus and cancer: the epidemiological evidence. *J Clin Virol. 2000 Oct; 19 (1-2): 1-5.* https://pubmed.ncbi.nlm.nih.gov/11091013/

Najib, F.S., et al. (2020). Diagnostic accuracy of cervical Pap smear and colposcopy in detecting premalignant and malignant lesions of cervix. *Indian J Surg Oncol. 2020 Sep; 11 (3): 453-458.* https://pubmed.ncbi.nlm.nih.gov/33013127/

Nicolas, F., et al. (2013). Are vaginal Pap smears necessary after total hysterectomy for CIN-3? *Gynecol Obstet Fertil. 2013 Mar; 41 (3): 196-200.* https://pubmed.ncbi.nlm.nih.gov/23499311/

Optimox. (2022). *Optimox.* Optimox: South Salt Lake, Utah. Retrieved 3 July 2022 https://www.optimox.com

Ouhoummane, N., et al. (2013). Squamous anal cancer: patient characteristics and HPV type distribution. *Cancer Epidemiol. 2013 Dec; 37 (6): 807-12.* https://pubmed.ncbi.nlm.nih.gov/24139594/

Panahi, Y., et al. (2015). Efficacy and safety of *Aloe vera* syrup for the treatment of gastroesophageal reflux disease: a pilot randomized positive-controlled trial. *J Tradit Chin Med. 2015 Dec; 35 (6): 632-6.* https://pubmed.ncbi.nlm.nih.gov/26742306/

Pessah-Pollack, R., et al. (2014). Apparent insufficiency of iodine supplementation in pregnancy. *J Womens Health (Larchmt). 2014 Jan; 23 (1): 51-6.* https://pubmed.ncbi.nlm.nih.gov/24117002/

Piscitelli, J.T., et al. (1995). Cytologic screening after hysterectomy for benign disease. *Am J Obstet Gynecol. 1995 Aug; 173 (2): 424-30; discussion 430-2.* https://pubmed.ncbi.nlm.nih.gov/7645617/

Plantz, M.A., et al. (2022). Dietary Calcium. Treasure Island, Florida:

StatPearls Publishing. May 22, 2022. https://www.ncbi.nlm.nih.gov/books/NBK549792/

Poljak, M., et al. (2020). Commercially available molecular tests for human papillomaviruses: a global overview. *Clin Microbiol Infect. 2020 Sep; 26 (9): 1144-1150.* https://pubmed.ncbi.nlm.nih.gov/32247892/

Puranen, M., et al. (1996). Transmission of genital human papillomavirus infections is unlikely through the floor and seats of humid dwellings in countries of high-level hygiene. *Scand J Infect Dis. 1996; 28 (3): 243-6.* https://pubmed.ncbi.nlm.nih.gov/8863354/

Qian, M., et al. (2005). The effects of iodine on intelligence in children: a meta-analysis of studies conducted in China. *Asia Pac J Clin Nutr. 2005; 14 (1): 32-42.* https://pubmed.ncbi.nlm.nih.gov/15734706/

Radu, M.C., et al. (2021). Human papillomavirus infection at the time of delivery. *Cureus. 2021 Jun 1; 13 (6): e15364.* https://pubmed.ncbi.nlm.nih.gov/34094788/

Rahangdale, L., et al. (2014). Topical 5-fluorouracil for treatment of cervical intraepithelial neoplasia 2: a randomized controlled trial. *Am J Obstet Gynecol. 2014 Apr; 210 (4): 314.e1-314.e8.* https://pubmed.ncbi.nlm.nih.gov/24384495/

Rappaport, J. (2017). Changes in dietary iodine explains increasing incidence of breast cancer with distant involvement in young women. *J Cancer. 2017; 8 (2): 174–177.* https://www.ncbi.nlm.nih.gov/pmc/articles/PMC5327366/

Rice, P.S., et al. (1999). High-risk genital papillomavirus infections are spread vertically. *Rev Med Virol. Jan-Mar 1999; 9 (1): 15-21.* https://pubmed.ncbi.nlm.nih.gov/10371668/

Richardson, H., et al. (2000). Determinants of low-risk and high-risk cervical human papillomavirus infections in Montreal University students. *Sex Transm Dis. 2000 Feb; 27 (2): 79-86.* https://pubmed.ncbi.nlm.nih.gov/10676974/

Bibliography

Riis, J., et al. (2021). Long-term iodine nutrition is associated with longevity in older adults: a 20 years' follow-up of the Randers-Skagen study. *Br J Nutr. 2021 Feb 14; 125 (3): 260-265.* https://pubmed.ncbi.nlm.nih.gov/32378500/

Sand, L., et al. (2000). Human papillomaviruses in oral lesions. *Anticancer Res. Mar-Apr 2000; 20 (2B): 1183-8.* https://pubmed.ncbi.nlm.nih.gov/10810419/

Schiffman, M.H., et al. (1993). Epidemiologic evidence showing that human papillomavirus infection causes most cervical intraep ithelial neoplasia. *J Natl Cancer Inst. 1993 Jun 16; 85 (12): 958-64.* https://pubmed.ncbi.nlm.nih.gov/8388478/

Schomburg, L., et al. (2008). On the importance of selenium and iodine metabolism for thyroid hormone biosynthesis and human health. *Mol Nutr Food Res. 2008 Nov; 52 (11): 1235-46.* https://pubmed.ncbi.nlm.nih.gov/18686295/

Segovia, Andrea. (2022). *The Natural Cure for HPV. pp. 15-24.* Retrieved 3 July 2022 https://bit.ly/naturalcureforhpv

Sellors, J.W., et al. (2003). Incidence, clearance, and predictors of human papillomavirus infection in women. *CMAJ. 2003 Feb 18; 168 (4): 421-5.* https://pubmed.ncbi.nlm.nih.gov/12591782/

Serth, J., et al. (1999). Increased levels of human papillomavirus type 16 DNA in a subset of prostate cancers. *Cancer Res 1999 Feb 15; 59 (4): 823-5.* https://pubmed.ncbi.nlm.nih.gov/10029070/

Sherman, M.E., et al. (1994). Toward objective quality assurance in cervical cytopathology. Correlation of cytopathologic diagnoses with detection of high-risk human papillomavirus types. *Am J Clin Pathol. 1994 Aug; 102 (2): 182-7.* https://pubmed.ncbi.nlm.nih.gov/8042586/

Shigehara, K., et al. (2010). Prevalence of human papillomavirus infection in the urinary tract of men with urethritis. *Int J Urol. 2010 Jun; 17 (6): 563-8.* https://pubmed.ncbi.nlm.nih.gov/20345431/

Shlisky, J., et al. (2022). Calcium deficiency worldwide: prevalence of inadequate intakes and associated health outcomes. *Ann N Y Acad Sci. 2022 Jun; 1512 (1): 10-28.* https://pubmed.ncbi.nlm.nih.gov/35247225/

Sichero, L., et al. (2019). Human papillomavirus and genital disease in men: what we have learned from the HIM study. *Acta Cytol. 2019; 63 (2): 109-117.* https://pubmed.ncbi.nlm.nih.gov/30799416/

Siegler, E., et al. (2017). The prevalence of HPV types in women with CIN 2-3 or cervical cancer in Haifa District, Israel. *Minerva Ginecol. 2017 Jun; 69 (3): 211-217.* https://pubmed.ncbi.nlm.nih.gov/27636902/

Sikstrom, B., et al. (1997). Gynecological symptoms and vaginal wet smear findings in women with cervical human papillomavirus infection. *Gynecol Obstet Invest. 1997; 43 (1): 49-52.* https://pubmed.ncbi.nlm.nih.gov/9015700/

Singh, V., et al. (1995). Clinical presentation of gynecologic infections among Indian women. *Obstet Gynecol. 1995 Feb; 85 (2): 215-9.* https://pubmed.ncbi.nlm.nih.gov/7824233/

Singh, V., et al. (1999). Biological behavior and etiology of inflammatory cervical smears. *Diagn Cytopathol. 1999 Apr; 20 (4): 199-202.* https://pubmed.ncbi.nlm.nih.gov/10204101/

Smith, J.A., et al. (2019). From bench to bedside: evaluation of AHCC supplementation to modulate the host immunity to clear high-risk human papillomavirus infections. *Front Oncol. 2019 Mar 20; 9: 173.* https://pubmed.ncbi.nlm.nih.gov/30949451/

Smith, J.A., et al. (2022). AHCC® supplementation to support immune function to clear persistent human papillomavirus infections. *Front Oncol. 2022 Jun 22; 12: 881902.* https://pubmed.ncbi.nlm.nih.gov/35814366/

Sonnex, C., et al. (1999). Detection of human papillomavirus DNA on the fingers of patients with genital warts. *Sex Transm Infect. 1999 Oct; 75 (5): 317-9.* https://pubmed.ncbi.nlm.nih.gov/10616355/

Sonnex, C., et al. (1999). Pearly penile papules: a common cause of concern. *Int J STD AIDS. 1999 Nov; 10 (11): 726-7.* https://pubmed. ncbi.nlm.nih.gov/10563558/

Spierings, E.L.H., et al. (2007). A Phase I study of the safety of the nutritional supplement, active hexose correlated compound, AHCC, in healthy volunteers. *J Nutr Sci Vitaminol (Tokyo). 2007; Dec; 53 (6): 536-9.* https://pubmed.ncbi.nlm.nih.gov/18202543/

Stanley, M. (1998). The immunology of genital human papillomavirus infection. *Eur J Dermatol. Oct-Nov 1998; 8 (7 Suppl): 8-12;* https://pubmed.ncbi.nlm.nih.gov/

Steele, K., et al. (1988). A study of HPV 1, 2, and 4 antibody prevalence in patients presenting for treatment with cutaneous warts to general practitioners in *N. Ireland. Epidemiol Infect. 1988 Dec; 101 (3): 537-46.* https://pubmed.ncbi.nlm.nih.gov/2850937/

Storsrud, S., et al. (2015). A pilot study of the effect of *Aloe barbadensis miller* extract (AVH200®) in patients with irritable bowel syndrome: A randomized, double-blind, placebo-controlled study. *J Gastrointestin Liver Dis. 2015 Sep; 24 (3): 275-80.* https:// pubmed.ncbi.nlm.nih.gov/26405698/

Strand, A., et al. (1998). Human papillomavirus. Subclinical and atypical manifestations. *Dermatol Clin. 1998 Oct; 16 (4): 817-22.* https://pubmed.ncbi.nlm.nih.gov/9891687/

Sun, Z., et al. (2018). *Aloe* polysaccharides inhibit influenza A virus infection—a promising natural anti-flu drug. *Front Microbiol. 2018; 9: 2338.* https://www.ncbi.nlm.nih.gov/pmc/articles/PMC6170609/

Surjushe, A., et al. (2008). *Aloe vera:* a short review. *Indian J Dermatol. 2008; 53 (4): 163–166.* https://www.ncbi.nlm.nih.gov/pmc/arti cles/PMC2763764/

Suzuki, H., et al. (1996). Detection of human papillomavirus DNA and p53 gene mutations in human prostate cancer. *Prostate. 1996 May; 28 (5): 318-24.* https://pubmed.ncbi.nlm.nih.gov/8610059/

Swiderska-Kiec, J., et al. (2020). Comparison of HPV testing and colposcopy in detecting cervical dysplasia in patients with cyto-

Bibliography

logical abnormalities. *In Vivo. May-Jun 2020; 34 (3): 1307-1315.* https://pubmed.ncbi.nlm.nih.gov/32354923/

Tanaka, M., et al. (2016). Effects of *Aloe* sterol supplementation on skin elasticity, hydration, and collagen score: A 12-week double-blind, randomized, controlled trial. *Skin Pharmacol Physiol. 2016; 29 (6): 309-317.* https://pubmed.ncbi.nlm.nih.gov/28088806/

Tenti, P., et al. (1999). Perinatal transmission of human papillomavirus from gravidas with latent infections. *Obstet Gynecol. 1999 Apr; 93 (4): 475-9.* https://pubmed.ncbi.nlm.nih.gov/10214817/

Toliopoulos, I., et al. (2012). NK cell stimulation by administration of vitamin C and *Aloe vera* juice in vitro and in vivo: A pilot study. *J Herbal Medicine. 2012 June; 2 (2): 29-33.* https://www.sciencedirect.com/science/article/abs/pii/S2210803312000371

Turner, M.L., and Marinoff, S.C. (1988). Association of human papillomavirus with vulvodynia and the vulvar vestibulitis syndrome. *J Reprod Med. 1988 Jun; 33 (6): 533-7.* https://pubmed.ncbi.nlm.nih.gov/2841460/

Valeix, P., et al. (1994). Relationship between urinary iodine concentration and hearing capacity in children. *Eur J Clin Nutr. 1994 Jan; 48 (1): 54-9.* https://pubmed.ncbi.nlm.nih.gov/8200329/

Van Den Briel, T., et al. (2000). Improved iodine status is associated with improved mental performance of school children in Benin. *Am J Clin Nutr. 2000 Nov; 72 (5): 1179-85.* https://pubmed.ncbi.nlm.nih.gov/11063446/

Videlefsky, A., et al. (2000). Routine vaginal cuff smear testing in post-hysterectomy patients with benign uterine conditions: when is it indicated? *J Am Board Fam Pract. Jul-Aug 2000; 13 (4): 233-8.* https://pubmed.ncbi.nlm.nih.gov/10933286/

Vitals Consumer Services LLC. (2022). *MedHelp: HPV, Cone Biopsy, Children, Beta-mannan™.* Vitals Consumer Services LLC: San Francisco, California. Retrieved 3 July 2022 https://www.medhelp.org/posts/Womens-Health/HPV-Cone-Biopsy-Chil

dren-Beta-mannan-and-now-new-problem-What-to-do/show/ 26690

Vives, A., et al. (2020). The role of human papillomavirus test in men: First exhaustive review of literature. *Actas Urol Esp (Engl Ed)*. *2020 Mar; 44 (2): 86-93.* https://pubmed.ncbi.nlm.nih.gov/ 31874781/

Wang, K., et al. (2018). Severely low serum magnesium is associated with increased risks of positive anti-thyroglobulin antibody and hypothyroidism: A cross-sectional study. *Sci Rep. 2018; 8: 9904.* https://www.ncbi.nlm.nih.gov/pmc/articles/PMC6028657/

Williams, S. (2018). *The Motley Fool: The cost of developing an FDA-approved drug is truly staggering, studies show.* The Motley Fool: Alexandria, Virginia. Retrieved 3 July 2022 https://www.fool. com/investing/general/2016/04/30/the-cost-of-developing-an-fda-approved-drug-is-tru.aspx

Winer, R.L., et al. (2003). Genital human papillomavirus infection: incidence and risk factors in a cohort of female university students. *Am J Epidemiol. 2003 Feb 1; 157 (3): 218-26.* https:// pubmed.ncbi.nlm.nih.gov/12543621/

Yao, X., et al. (2021). Naturally acquired HPV antibodies against subsequent homotypic infection: A large-scale prospective cohort study. *Lancet Reg Health West Pac. 2021 Aug; 13: 100196.* https://pubmed.ncbi.nlm.nih.gov/34527987/

Yin, B., et al. (2017). Association between human papillomavirus and prostate cancer: A meta-analysis. *Oncol Lett. 2017 Aug; 14 (2): 1855–1865.* https://www.ncbi.nlm.nih.gov/pmc/articles/ PMC5529902/

Yu, H., et al. (2002). Molecular biological study of *Aloe vera* in the treatment of experimental allergic rhinitis in the rat. *Lin Chuang Er Bi Yan Hou Ke Za Zhi. 2002 May; 16 (5): 229-31.* https:// pubmed.ncbi.nlm.nih.gov/12592663/

Yuan, S., et al. (2019). Human papillomavirus infection and female infertility: a systematic review and meta-analysis. *Reprod Biomed*

Online. *2020 Feb; 40 (2): 229-237.* https://pubmed.ncbi.nlm.nih.gov/31987733/

Zhang, C., et al. (2017). Incidence and clearance of oral human papillomavirus infection: A population-based cohort study in rural China. *Oncotarget.* *2017 Aug 29; 8 (35): 59831–59844.* https://www.ncbi.nlm.nih.gov/pmc/articles/PMC5601782/

Zhang, Y., et al. (2016). Efficacy of *Aloe vera* supplementation on pre-diabetes and early non-treated diabetic patients: A systematic review and meta-analysis of randomized controlled trials. *Nutrients.* *2016 Jul; 8 (7): 388.* https://www.ncbi.nlm.nih.gov/pmc/articles/PMC4963864/

About the Author

C.W. Willington is a medical writer fascinated by our immune system's response to viruses.

Made in United States
Orlando, FL
14 January 2024

42514698R00183